Antonio Marcos Moreira Aguilar
Monia Maia Lima

Leprosy

Antonio Marcos Moreira Aguilar
Monia Maia Lima

Leprosy

Geospatial Behaviour in the State of Mato Grosso

ScienciaScripts

Imprint

Cover image: www.ingimage.com

This book is a translation from the original published under ISBN 978-613-9-69684-0.

Publisher:
Sciencia Scripts
is a trademark of
Dodo Books Indian Ocean Ltd. and OmniScriptum S.R.L publishing group

120 High Road, East Finchley, London, N2 9ED, United Kingdom
Str. Armeneasca 28/1, office 1, Chisinau MD-2012, Republic of Moldova, Europe
Printed at: see last page
ISBN: 978-620-8-13444-0

I dedicate this work

To my wife Mônia Maia de Lima, for her support and patience during the course of this work.

ACKNOWLEDGEMENTS

To my parents, Joaquim Costa Aguilar and Maria Emília Moreira Aguilar, references in my life of character, simplicity and courage.

To my siblings, Reinaldo Moreira Aguilar, Mônica Moreira Aguilar and Reginaldo Moreira Aguilar, for their loyalty and companionship.

To God, for never forgetting me in moments of instability, being present in every situation in my life.

To Dr Wagner Izidoro de Brito, for his patience and relevant collaboration in carrying out this work.

Dr Adriana Zilly, for her guidance and technical support in the development of this research.

To Mr Luciano de Andrade, for his commitment and dedication throughout this process.

"In Memoriam
To my mentor Dr Carlos Alberto Faria Rodrigues, for fostering in me the ability to strive to be the best, not only in leprosy, but in all aspects of being human. May you be at God's side and help me along this long road. Thank you for your dedication and for all your teachings.

"Every man afflicted with leprosy shall have his clothes torn and his head uncovered. He shall cover his beard and cry, 'Unclean! Unclean!'" (Leviticus)

SUMMARY

The aim of this study was to analyse the geospatial behaviour of leprosy in the state of Mato Grosso. An ecological, cross-sectional study was carried out using secondary data from DATASUS, SINAN and TABNET, from 2007 to 2011. The study site was the Epidemiological Surveillance Department of the municipality of Primavera do Leste - MT. Once the database had been prepared, it was analysed using the GEODA software (ANSELIN, 2005), version 0.9.5, Spatial Analysis Laboratory, University of Illinois at Urbana-Champaign, Urbana, United States, using the Global Moran's Index, uni- and bivariate analysis, in order to assess the autocorrelation between morbidity rates and socioeconomic and demographic variables. Epidemiological clusters were also produced, as well as Moran's scatter plots. The results showed that the state of Mato Grosso is endemic for leprosy. During the period observed, 13,648 cases were recorded, with a predominance of cases in the 40-69 age group. The prevalence within the 141 municipalities is high, exceeding 16 cases / 10,000 inhabitants, well above that recommended by the Ministry of Health. The univariate analysis for children under fifteen showed positive spatial autocorrelation (I=0.220711 p= 0.001), demonstrating that areas with high rates of leprosy cases are surrounded by municipalities with the same epidemiological characteristics. The clusters showed areas with a high number of records, corroborating the state's condition at national level. With regard to socioeconomic and demographic variables, the illiteracy rate was positive (p=0.011), as was the gini coefficient (p=0.020), showing that both influence the vulnerability of a given population to falling ill with leprosy. However, the variables income (p=0.063) and demographic density (p=0.365) resulted in spatial independence and were not relevant predisposing factors. It can be concluded that the state of Mato Grosso accounts for a significant proportion of leprosy cases in Brazil. Throughout its territory, the disease is present in high numbers. The disease in children under fifteen is worrying, as this indicator is the Ministry of Health's main tool for assessing the behaviour of this pathology. Focusing on educational actions and reducing social inequalities are priorities for reducing these numbers in the long term.

Key words: Leprosy. Public Health. Epidemiology

SUMMARY

CHAPTER 1

INTRODUCTION

The social image of leprosy is historical. The development of science was not enough to change the response of fear and prejudice towards the disease, despite Armanuer Hansen, at the end of the 19th century, discovering the causative agent of the disease, proving its infectious nature and cancelling out the idea of heredity, sin or punishment, the theory still emerged that isolating the patient would eliminate the disease, encouraging the adoption of a treatment model based on the restriction of freedom in large isolation institutions. To this day, the impact caused by the disease interferes in the daily lives of individuals, who have leprosy as a constant threat of prejudice marked by suffering, abandonment, deformities and psychosocial problems (BOTI; AQUINO, 2008).

It is very difficult to say when a disease first appeared on the basis of ancient texts, unless there is a reasonable description of the illness, citing its most characteristic aspects. If this is not the case, and if we rely only on fragmentary data and assumptions made by translators of those texts, the subject becomes confusing and generates a series of false interpretations with sometimes unpredictable consequences (OPROMOLLA, 2000).

Hansen's disease (HM) continues to be a serious public health problem and is endemic in several countries around the world. It is mainly characterised by neurological and dermatological manifestations that lead to deformities and mutilations after a long period of time (VERONESI and FOCACCIA, 2009, p. 1055).

The leprosy hyperendemic found in many municipalities in the study area was in common with the findings of other authors and, when associated with operational factors, suggests a "hidden incidence" of the disease. This suggests that part of the transcendence of the endemic is due to a lack of diagnosis (SOUZA, 2012).

Considering the growing epidemiology of leprosy in the state of Mato Grosso, this study takes on important scientific characteristics and aims to contribute to discussions at the level of society as well as management, with regard to the prevalence of this disease in the state.

CHAPTER 2

LITERATURE REVIEW

2.1 HISTORICAL ASPECTS

The tropical and subtropical belt of Africa and southern Asia are considered to be the ancestral cradle of leprosy, where evidence of the disease dates back more than 2,500 years. Until the 19th century, leprosy was endemic in regions as far north as the Arctic Circle. In northern Europe the disease spread 1,000 years ago. Its prevalence was on the rise until the 13th century, then gradually declined until it disappeared (QUEIROZ, 2009).

Its disappearance from northern Europe remains one of the greatest enigmas of its epidemiology, and various causes are attributed to this fact: improved socio-economic conditions and living standards; better nutrition; effective isolation of infectious cases; genetic selection of the population; inhibitory competition with other mycobacteria, especially Mycobacterium tuberculosis; selective mortality of leprosy patients during plague epidemics (QUEIROZ, 2009).

The existence of this disease in ancient times is reported in many other regions, but the data is confusing (OPROMOLLA, 2000). The possibility of a multifocal origin of the disease cannot be ruled out a priori. The disease may have been transmitted to the Egyptians by the Hebrew pilgrims (VERONESI and FOCACCIA, 2009).

The oldest and most accurate descriptions of MH come from India, 600 years BC (Indian Medical Treatise of Sushrata Samhita calls it "Kushta"). According to traditions passed down verbally, this illness was already mentioned 6,000 years before our era. The descriptions of Leviticus in the Bible refer to it as far back as 1400 BC (VERONESI and FOCACCIA, 2009, p.1047).

According to Sampaio and Rivitti (2007, p. 625), the time when leprosy first appeared is not known. In ancient history, BC, there are descriptions compatible with leprosy in Chinese and Hindu texts.

In Brazil, the first documents attesting to the existence of leprosy in our territory date back to the end of the 17th century, so much so that in 1696, Governor Artur de Sá e Menezes sought to provide assistance in Rio de Janeiro to the "miserable lepers", who were already in appreciable numbers (OPROMOLLA, 2000).

The initial source and prehistoric transmission routes of "leprosy" are not unanimous either, and have long been attributed to the Old World. The three most ancient civilisations of humanity - Indian, Egyptian and Hebrew - have been blamed. Ancient reports and signs of the disease on Indian skeletons and Egyptian mummies are a source of controversy, and the most widely accepted probability is that "leprosy" originated on the Indian subcontinent and was introduced to Europe by Alexander the Great's troops. Another possibility is that there are two currents of the disease: Asian and African (MONOT et al, 2005).

Leprosy was already well known around 150 AD, when we find references to it by Areteus of Cappadocia and Galen (OPROMOLLA, 2000). The first author in his work "Therapeutics of Chronic Ailments" calls leprosy Elephas or Elephantiasis and says that "there are many things in common as regards shape, colour, size and way of life between the Elephas affection and the wild beast, the elephant, and neither does this affection resemble any other affection, nor the animal any other animal" (OPROMOLLA, 2000).

Later on, he talks about the similarity between the condition of the skin in the disease and the skin of an elephant. It was he who first called the infiltrated face of patients with leprosy "leonine face" (OPROMOLLA, 2000).

However, leprosy was referred to as leprosy, as were all the diseases that were thought to be identical or related to it (OPROMOLLA, 2000). Another of the most authentic descriptions of leprosy in Chinese literature is the work "Complete Secret Remedies" written by Hua T'o (AMARAL, 2006).

Pompey's Roman legions, passing through Egypt in 61 BC, are believed to have taken leprosy to Italy and spread it throughout Europe (SOBRINHO, 2007). During the colonisation of the Americas, particularly Brazil, leprosy was introduced by European Portuguese immigrants and also by Africans, and over the years Latin America became an endemic area (SOBRINHO, 2007).

> In Brazil, the first cases of the disease were diagnosed in the 1600s, in the city of Rio de Janeiro, where the first leprosaria were set up. After the first cases in this state, other outbreaks of the disease were identified, mainly in Bahia and Pará (SOBRINHO, 2007).

In its magnitude, the process of spreading this disease globally can be associated with factors such as: agglomerations, poor socio-economic conditions, the lack of diagnostic processes, nutritional, cultural, migratory and climatic factors.

> The disease was very prevalent in Europe between 1000 and 1400 AD. The Vikings, coming from England in the 11th century, infected the Scandinavians. In the 12th and 13th centuries, the disease existed in violent expansion, it was a true pandemic throughout Europe. The endemic spread, especially among the soldiers of the Crusades and merchants (VERONESI and FOCACCIA, 2009, p. 1048).

It is clear that a large part of the stigma generated by this disease is due much more to prejudice than to the objective condition of the disease, since the vast majority of individuals offer immunological resistance to Mycobacterium leprae, the causative agent of the disease (QUEIROZ; PUNTEL, 1997). Waxier develops this thesis, showing various cultural situations with positively or negatively charged attitudes towards stigma in the manifestation of leprosy (QUEIROZ; PUNTEL,

1997). Patients were also obliged to wear characteristic clothing that identified them as such and to ring a bell or nunchaku to warn the healthy of their approach (QUEIROZ; PUNTEL, 1997).

2.2 EPIDEMIOLOGY

Between 2001 and 2003, 18,976.93 cases of leprosy were recorded worldwide, with the Southeast Asian region predominating, with 15,948.99. This data reinforces this pathology as a serious public health problem, making it imperative that the major powers articulate actions and targets for the global reduction of the disease transmission process (WHO, 2004).

According to Brasil (2008), worldwide leprosy data shows a reduction in the bacillary load in several countries, although health units, institutions and non-governmental organisations are aware of its growing incidence. N detection (rate/100,000 inhabitants) was 249,007 cases, with the Southeast Asian region predominating, with 167,505 (9.60 - 100,000 inhabitants), followed by the Americas with 41,891 (4.85 - 100,000 inhabitants), Africa with 29,814 cases (4.37 - 100,000 inhabitants), the Western Pacific with 5,859 (0.33 - 100,000 inhabitants) and the Eastern Mediterranean with 3,938 cases (0.80 - 100,000 inhabitants). 94% of the patients notified were in Angola, Bangladesh, Brazil, China, Congo, India, Ethiopia, Indonesia, Madagascar, Mozambique, Myanmar, Nepal, Nigeria, Philippines, Sri Lanka, Sudan and Tanzania.

In Brazil, a comparative analysis between 2001-2007 revealed a reduction in incidence (per 100,000 inhabitants) in all regions of the country, with 54.25% of cases in the North, 31.53% in the Northeast, 40.65% in the Centre-West, 6.45% and 9.75% in the Southeast (MAINENTI, 2010). Brasil (2012) points to a 25.9 per cent reduction in new cases between 2001 and 2011, from 45,874 to 33,955, respectively. Despite the results, in 2011 seven states had a prevalence rate above three cases per 10,000 inhabitants (MT, TO, MA, PA, RO, GO, MS).

The national average is 1.54/10,000, which is very close to the target set by the Plan for the Elimination of Leprosy (less than one case per group of 10,000 inhabitants). Leprosy in the state of Mato Grosso has endemic characteristics. According to preliminary data from (BRASIL, 2011), the state had a prevalence rate of 7.52 / 10,000 inhabitants.

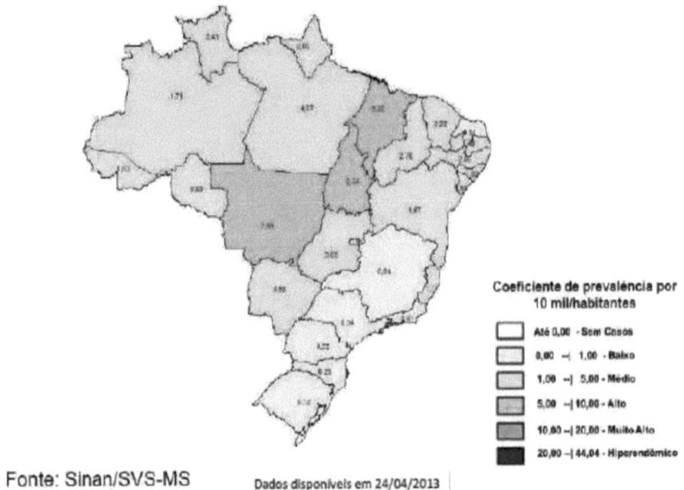

Figure 1 - HANSENIASIS PREVALENCE COEFFICIENT BY STATE BRAZIL - 2012.

Brasil (2010) also discusses these indicators, emphasising that the distribution of leprosy is very heterogeneous. In 2008, according to the National Notifiable Diseases System (SINAN), the country's detection coefficient was 20.59/100,000 inhabitants, with a total of 39,047 new cases recorded. In the same year, the detection coefficient in Rio Grande do Sul was 1.66/100,000 inhabitants and in Tocantins 103.63/100,000 inhabitants. The highest rate was recorded in the North (54.69/100,000 inhabitants) and the lowest in the South (6.05/100,000 inhabitants). The most prevalent regions (NORTH, NORTHEAST and CENTRE WEST) accounted for 77% of all new cases and 86.3% of cases reported in children under fifteen.

Every year, the Sasakawa Foundation (The Nippon Foundation) coordinates the signing by world leaders and organisations of a commitment called the Global Appeal. The aim is to strengthen the defence of a world without leprosy (BRASIL, 2012).

In 1985, the number of leprosy cases in the world, mainly in tropical regions, was estimated at between 13 and 14 million, with almost 5.5 million cases registered. Since the introduction by the WHO (World Health Organisation) of MDT (Multi-Drug Therapy) or TMM (Multi-Medication Therapy), adopted in Brazil under the name PQT (Polychemotherapy), there has been a surprising decrease in the endemic worldwide (SAMPAIO and RIVITTI, 2007).

It is a public health problem in many countries in Asia, Africa, Latin America and the Caribbean. According to a study carried out by the World Health Organisation (WHO) to detect new cases between 1985 and 2006, in 2001 the number of new cases detected by the WHO was 763,262. Since then, there has been a decrease in registrations, reaching 259,017 cases in 2006. However, in the region of the Americas, there has been an increase in the number of new cases per year, so that between 1991 and 2006, 47,612 cases were diagnosed, 93 per cent of them in Brazil. Due to the large variations in regional prevalence coefficients, the country's epidemiological situation was considered heterogeneous (PINTO et al, 2010).

Compared to neighbouring Latin American countries, Brazil has the highest incidence and prevalence rates, considering, of course, Brazil's geodemographic size compared to other countries. In Uruguay, in December 1988, the prevalence coefficient reached 0.99 per 10,000 inhabitants, i.e. national elimination was achieved. In December 1998, with a national prevalence coefficient of 0.04 per 10,000 inhabitants, elimination was achieved at sub-national level. In 2001, the national detection coefficient was 0.38 per 10,000 inhabitants, with 12 new cases detected. The current leprosy situation in Uruguay is a post-elimination scenario with sporadic cases in various departments (PAHO, 2002).

In Cuba, elimination at national level was achieved in 1993 with a coefficient of 0.79 per 10,000 inhabitants. At the end of 2001, of all 15 provinces, only one had a prevalence coefficient of more than 1 per 10,000 inhabitants. There has been a reduction in the percentage of cases detected with advanced disability (grade 2) from 5% in 1996 to 3.4% in 2001 (PAHO, 2002).

As far as Paraguay is concerned, the distribution of leprosy incidence and prevalence is uniform throughout the country. The prevalence coefficient is less than 1 per 10,000 inhabitants at national level and, in recent years, the detection coefficient has remained constant at 0.82 per 10,000 inhabitants. There is a large component of activities carried out by NGOs (Hospital Mennonita Km 81, DAHW), aimed at integrating leprosy care into the basic health system. In 2001, the country registered the lowest prevalence coefficient, 0.93 per 10,000 inhabitants, which represented the achievement of the goal of eliminating leprosy as a public health problem at national level, as well as having managed to detect a number of new cases totalling 467 (PAHO, 2002).

According to Brasil (2007), 210,800 new cases of leprosy were diagnosed and in the state of Bahia, for the same year, the estimated prevalence was 208,800 cases. The disease can be highly disabling and deforming, and the discrimination suffered by these patients and their families can make diagnosis difficult. When not diagnosed and treated early, leprosy can develop into deformities and disabilities. The sequelae left by the lesions are well defined and can be found from the moment of diagnosis. Studies show that it is difficult for local services in some regions to diagnose leprosy cases early, which can lead to an "epidemiological silence", delaying its elimination and effective control of the disease (PINTO et al, 2010).

In Brazil, as a result of the policies adopted by the Ministry of Health, there was a reduction in the number of cases from 19 to approximately five per 10,000 inhabitants between 1985 and 1999. However, the rate accepted by the World Health Organisation, i.e. less than one case per 10,000 inhabitants, has still not been achieved (DESSUNTI et al, 2008).

Brasil (2010) corroborates the endemic condition of leprosy in Brazil. In 2009, 36,718 new cases were reported, with a detection rate of 19.18/100,000 inhabitants. In the case of children under fifteen, 2,617 cases were reported, with a detection rate of 5.33/100,000 inhabitants, well above that recommended by the World Health Organisation (WHO). From an epidemiological point of view, 57% of the patients belonged to the multibacillary forms, with males predominating (55.2%).

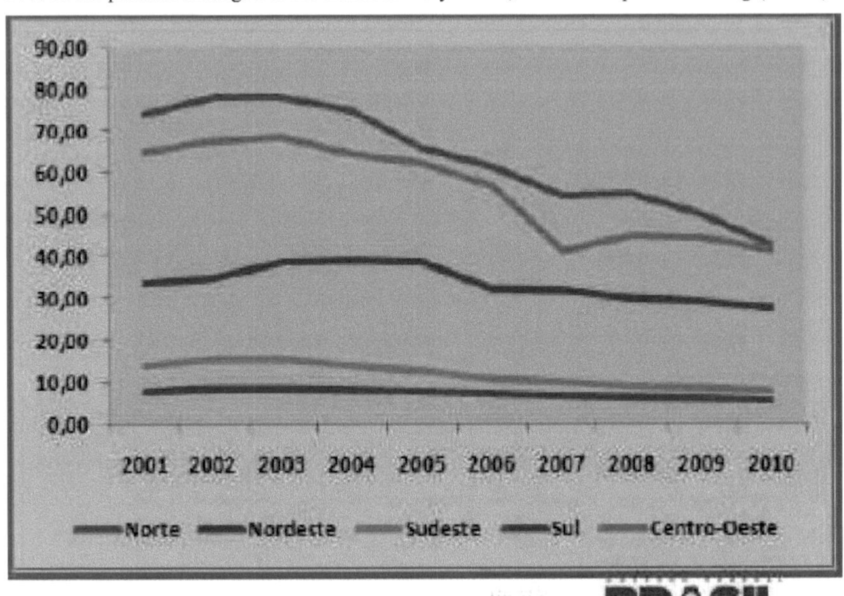

GRAPH 1 - GENERAL DETECTION COEFFICIENT OF HANSENIASIS BY FEDERAL UNIT, BRAZIL, 2001 to 2010.

In line with Mainenti (2010), a comparative analysis between 2001 and 2007 revealed a reduction in incidence (per 100,000 inhabitants) in all regions of the country, with 54.25% of cases in the North, 31.53% in the Northeast, 40.65% in the Centre West, 6.45% in the South and 9.75% in the Southeast. Leprosy is showing a trend of stabilisation in the detection coefficients in Brazil. However, it is very high in the North, Centre West and Northeast.

In 2005, the prevalence coefficient fell to 1.48 cases per 10,000 inhabitants, equivalent to 27,313 people being treated. The detection rate was 2.09 per 10,000 inhabitants, corresponding to the notification of 38,410 cases. However, Brazil has maintained an average of 47,000 new cases per year over the last five years (DESSUNTI et al, 2008).

After a retrospective study, Araújo (2003) corroborated Brazil's position as the second country in terms of the number of cases in the world. Approximately 94% of known cases in the Americas and 94% of diagnosed cases are notified by Brazil. Paradoxically, while prevalence rates showed a quantitative decline, new case detection rates remained high, thus delaying the goal of eliminating the disease.

Some principles stand out in the elimination of leprosy: control of morbidity, timely detection of new cases, treatment in the form of appropriate MDT, prevention of disabilities and rehabilitation of leprosy patients. Given their effectiveness in controlling the endemic, these principles are unlikely to change in the coming years (WHO, 2005).

Queiroz (1997) says that the growth of the endemic is also linked to factors such as incomplete diagnosis, unpreparedness on the part of health professionals in terms of care (treatment of the sick, control and monitoring of communicants) and education (group work, lectures, home visits) aimed at preventing the disease. Prejudice on the part of health professionals is also a barrier to the development of a control programme for patients and their contacts. It has been agreed that leprosy is a major health problem whenever the prevalence of the disease is greater than 1 case per 1,000 inhabitants.

Areas with coefficients of less than 0.2 cases per thousand inhabitants are considered to be of low endemicity, while coefficients between 0.2 and 1.0 per thousand inhabitants correspond to areas of medium endemicity. In a region of high endemicity, the risk of contracting the disease increases in underdeveloped countries and regions, due to the poor coverage of health services and unprepared technical staff (QUEIROZ, 1997).

TABLE 1: GENERAL DETECTION COEFFICIENT OF HANSENIASIS PER 100,000 HABITANT STATES AND REGIONS, BRAZIL, 2001 to 2012.

Coeficiente de detecção geral de hanseníase por 100.000 habitantes
Estados e regiões, Brasil, 2001 a 2012

Estados / regiões	2001	2002	2003	2004	2005	2006	2007	2008	2009	2010	2011	2012
Região Norte	**73,82**	**77,88**	**78,01**	**74,71**	**65,96**	**61,12**	**54,34**	**54,69**	**49,94**	**42,73**	**42,65**	**42,24**
Rondônia	82,46	84,37	96,71	90,68	82,76	85,96	73,96	70,44	69,49	58,76	53,98	51,13
Acre	70,16	61,50	66,60	51,94	54,05	76,75	39,38	39,26	37,76	34,53	30,55	23,46
Amazonas	43,45	48,18	37,78	34,16	29,76	25,61	22,96	21,01	21,54	19,71	16,59	18,49
Roraima	87,47	86,78	93,20	80,50	69,25	63,72	53,70	45,79	37,96	31,25	24,56	31,10
Pará	84,41	92,06	92,91	90,31	77,81	65,45	61,90	62,17	55,70	46,93	51,06	50,01
Amapá	28,47	35,82	37,21	33,45	27,92	30,05	19,63	31,15	30,32	21,53	24,70	21,76
Tocantins	98,24	90,72	94,21	100,54	95,04	102,67	93,53	103,71	88,54	77,92	70,74	73,43
Nordeste	**33,39**	**35,05**	**38,66**	**38,75**	**38,67**	**32,28**	**31,75**	**30,04**	**28,80**	**27,73**	**26,08**	**25,78**
Maranhão	80,94	86,76	87,54	90,28	92,00	73,39	69,75	67,34	61,99	60,46	56,11	55,54
Piauí	61,54	57,79	63,93	57,37	56,77	44,96	47,11	57,70	40,25	46,46	35,03	33,57
Ceará	34,70	32,84	37,58	34,67	34,76	29,07	30,17	29,62	26,16	25,34	23,00	24,82
Rio Grande do Norte	8,21	9,04	8,83	11,08	15,82	8,90	12,03	8,31	9,88	8,21	8,38	9,85
Paraíba	23,55	25,15	26,74	25,41	28,84	26,33	23,86	19,67	19,34	17,39	18,81	18,53
Pernambuco	39,03	41,23	44,14	40,69	39,51	37,61	35,93	31,95	36,45	31,78	30,02	27,66
Alagoas	12,95	14,03	17,96	14,89	14,95	14,32	13,61	12,57	12,86	12,10	12,76	14,41
Sergipe	17,33	23,67	31,85	28,95	33,54	25,84	26,02	22,31	24,51	18,42	20,77	22,55
Bahia	17,04	19,38	24,06	29,32	26,38	21,44	21,05	19,12	19,37	19,21	19,05	17,94

Região Sudeste	**14,06**	**15,32**	**15,14**	**13,84**	**12,60**	**10,53**	**9,76**	**8,78**	**8,42**	**7,66**	**7,42**	**6,60**
Minas Gerais	15,35	18,44	18,10	16,93	15,63	13,12	11,22	9,69	9,39	8,03	7,68	7,37
Espírito Santo	45,23	53,57	55,13	47,45	45,39	34,93	34,52	31,16	29,94	29,18	28,64	21,88
Rio de Janeiro	21,06	22,83	21,85	20,10	17,72	16,22	14,31	11,93	12,45	11,22	10,67	9,30
São Paulo	8,12	7,72	7,78	7,14	6,46	5,09	5,26	5,24	4,58	4,27	4,22	3,89
Região Sul	**7,44**	**8,50**	**8,42**	**7,96**	**7,57**	**6,99**	**6,44**	**6,05**	**5,54**	**5,19**	**4,99**	**4,83**
Paraná	15,60	17,61	17,39	16,02	15,47	14,54	13,06	12,09	11,17	10,19	9,63	9,35
Santa Catarina	3,43	3,98	4,17	4,19	3,70	3,51	3,62	3,39	3,04	3,38	3,61	3,20
Rio Grande do Sul	1,88	2,33	2,23	2,39	2,19	1,74	1,71	1,66	1,44	1,37	1,27	1,36
Região Centro-Oeste	**65,11**	**67,81**	**68,69**	**64,39**	**62,13**	**56,60**	**41,19**	**44,64**	**44,28**	**41,29**	**40,40**	**40,04**
Mato Grosso do Sul	26,95	28,54	32,59	31,93	27,34	27,11	23,81	26,93	27,92	26,62	29,75	34,97
Mato Grosso	146,26	140,71	144,49	131,07	136,45	125,13	100,13	87,97	89,48	81,64	85,37	80,34
Goiás	60,65	68,73	67,22	65,62	59,79	53,33	31,49	44,93	43,25	41,29	36,21	35,82
Distrito Federal	15,30	16,26	16,26	12,85	12,26	10,78	10,64	10,05	9,40	7,57	7,24	7,21
Brasil	**26,61**	**28,33**	**29,37**	**28,24**	**26,86**	**23,37**	**21,19**	**20,59**	**19,64**	**18,22**	**17,65**	**17,17**

Fonte: Sinan/SVS-MS Taxa por 100.000/habitantes Dados disponíveis em 24/04/2013

Nationwide, following an unprecedented study, Brasil (2012) points to a 25.9 per cent reduction in new cases between 2001 and 2011, from 45,874 to 33,955, respectively. Despite these results, in 2011 there were seven states with a prevalence coefficient above three cases per 10,000 inhabitants (MT, TO, MA, PA, RO, GO, MS). The national average is 1.54/10,000, which is very close to the target set by the Leprosy Elimination Plan (less than one case per group of 10,000 by 2015).

In Brazil, the Legal Amazon and the Centre-West and Northeast regions are the geographical areas responsible for the highest leprosy prevalence rates in the country. In 1997, the Legal Amazon had a prevalence rate of 15.5 cases per 10,000 inhabitants and a detection rate of 9.07 per 10,000. The Centre-West had a prevalence rate of 10.33 and a detection rate of 5.14, while the North-East had prevalence and detection rates of 4.73 and 2.41 cases per 10,000 inhabitants respectively. In 2003, the Northern region remained with the highest prevalence indicators in Brazil, contributing 15,764 cases of leprosy, which gave it a prevalence of 11.44 cases per 10,000 inhabitants, while the detection coefficient in the same year for the region was 7.61 cases per 10,000 inhabitants. The Centre-West region came second in terms of prevalence (8.75) and detection (6.54), followed by the Northeast region with a prevalence of 6.73 cases per 10,000 inhabitants and detection of 3.52 cases per 10,000 inhabitants (OLIVEIRA, 2008).

Notwithstanding the objectives proposed for such reductions, the federal programme listed 252 priority municipalities, determining a financial transfer of 16,515,000, with the commitment to expand efforts to eliminate leprosy as a public health problem (BRASIL, 2011).

It can be seen that Brazil has seen a drop in most epidemiological indicators over the last ten years, which reinforces the idea that access to basic services, early information and qualified professionals are important factors in this achievement. (PORTAL BRASIL, 2013) points out that the number of new cases of leprosy in children under 15 fell by 32% over the same period. In 2011, there were 2,420 cases and a detection coefficient of 5.2 per 100,000 inhabitants. In 2001, the coefficient was 6.96. The reduction can be explained by the expansion of treatment available in public health units, the increase in the capacity of professionals to carry out diagnoses, and also by the efforts of professionals in the basic network and reference centres. By 2015, the Ministry of Health aims to eliminate leprosy as a public health problem, which means achieving less than one case per 10,000 inhabitants. In 2011, Brazil registered 1.54 cases per 10,000 inhabitants, corresponding to 29,690 cases being treated.

TABLE 2 - LEPROSY PREVALENCE COEFFICIENT, GENERAL DETECTION AND DETECTION IN CHILDREN UNDER 15 BY REGION, BRAZIL 2011.

Leprosy prevalence rates, overall detection rates and detection rates in children under 15 by region, Brazil 2011

Region	Prevalence'	Parameters	Detection²	Parameters	New Cases <15 years	Coefficient <15 years'	Parameters
Northern Region	349	Medium	42,65	Hyper endemic	E7fi	13.34	Hyperendemic
North-East Region	2,35	Medium	26,08	Very high	1.166	8,10	Very high
South-East Region	061	Bass	7,42	Medium	276	1,58	Medium
Southern Region	0,44	Bass	4,99	Medium	20	0.33	Bass
Centre-West Region	3,75	Medium	40,40	Hypcrendemic	286	8,20	Very high
Brazil	1,54	Medium	17,65	High	2.420	5,22	Very high

Source: S"un'S/S-MS subtitle: 'Rate per 10,000 inhabitants Rate per tOO.OOOrhabitants Data available at 24042012

The figures are above the recommendations of international and national organisations. As it is the main indicator of the behaviour of the disease, the number of cases in children under fifteen deserves special attention from managers, technical teams and governments. (PIRES et al 2011) states that leprosy can affect all age groups, but reducing cases in children under 15 is a priority for the National Leprosy Control Programme (PNCH) of the Ministry of Health's Epidemiological Surveillance Secretariat, because when the disease manifests itself in childhood, especially in the zero to five age group, it indicates high endemicity, a lack of information about the disease in this age group and a lack of effective health education actions.

Barbierí and Marques (2009) point out that Brazil is responsible for 90% of cases on the American continent and is the second country in absolute number and incidence, registering around 47,000 new cases a year, second only to India. Within the country there are areas considered to be hyper-endemic, such as Mato Grosso and Roraima, and states where the disease is not endemic, such as Rio Grande do Sul, Santa Catarina and São Paulo.

The Brazilian Society of Dermatology (SBD, 2013) encourages discussions about the current epidemiology of leprosy in children under fifteen. It emphasises that reducing the number of leprosy cases in children under 15 is a priority in Brazil, as it is the main indicator for monitoring the endemic. Despite the fall in rates seen in recent years, 2,420 new cases were detected in this age group in 2011, which equated to a detection coefficient of 5.22 cases per 100,000 inhabitants. Leprosy in children indicates recent transmission through a nearby focus of active infection. Therefore, the high probability of finding the source of infection summarises the extreme importance of diagnosing leprosy in children under 15, which demonstrates the relevance of this initiative.

Leprosy can affect all age groups, but is more common in adults. The prevalence of the disease in children and adolescents under the age of 15 is higher in endemic countries, revealing the persistence of bacillus transmission and the difficulties health programmes face in controlling the disease. In India, it is believed that 20 to 25 per cent of cases are in children under 15. In Brazil, around 7 to 8 per cent of new cases are in children, corresponding to 0.6 cases per 10,000 inhabitants. However, the states of Mato Grosso, Maranhão, Tocantins, Roraima and Rondônia have a detection coefficient of more than 2 cases (in children under 15) per 10,000 inhabitants, which is considered high by the WHO (BARBIERI; MARQUES, 2009).

Leprosy in the state of Mato Grosso is endemic. According to preliminary data from BRASIL (2011), the state had a prevalence rate of 7.52/10,000 inhabitants, making it the leading state in the country.

Still within this context, the state of Mato Grosso is also ahead in terms of overall detection coefficients by federal unit, with 77.89/100,000 inhabitants. In terms of its position on the spectrum, Mato Grosso recorded a detection coefficient in children under fifteen of 17.96/100,000 inhabitants, taking second place in relation to the country's other federal units (BRASIL, 2011).

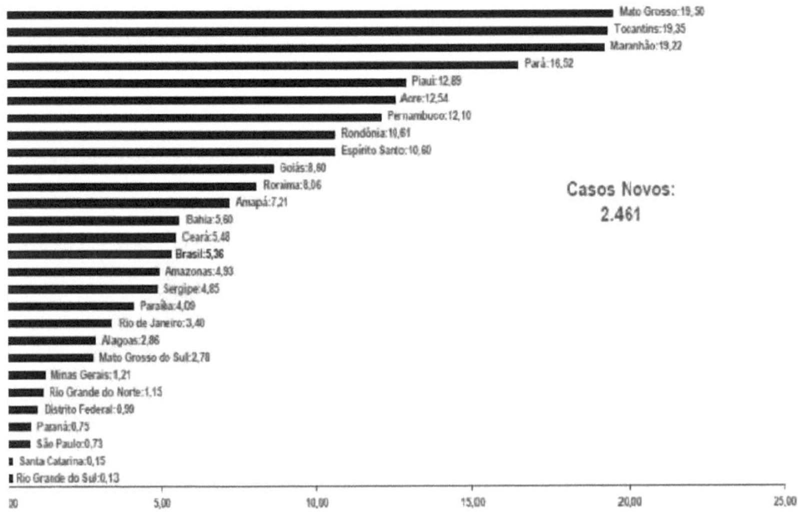

Graph 2 - DETECTION COEFFICIENT OF NEW CASES OF HANSENIASIS IN UNDER FIFTEEN YEARS OF AGE BRAZIL AND STATES, 2010.

With regard to this indicator, it can be seen that the state of Mato Grosso had the highest detection rate in Brazil, ahead of hyperendemic states such as Tocantins and Maranhão. (OLIVEIRA, 2008) shows that Ministry of Health data from 2005 reveals the need to focus on diagnosing leprosy in children under 15, who may be the contacts that have not yet been cared for or identified by the health system, so this is a very important action for subsequent strategies. It is clear that the municipalities are committed to discussing the elimination of leprosy, and that since the 1990s they have favoured the decentralisation of leprosy control activities.

CHAPTER 3

DEFINITION

Leprosy is an infectious, chronic disease of great importance to public health due to its magnitude and high incapacitating power, mainly affecting the economically active age group (BRASIL, 2008).

It is a chronic, granulomatous disease caused by infection with Mycobacterium Leprae. This bacillus has the ability to infect a large number of people.

These properties depend on the intrinsic characteristics of the bacillus, its relationship with the host and the degree of endemicity of the environment (BRASIL, 2010).

There are various theories about how the disease is transmitted. The most widely accepted hypothesis is that a person who is sick with the contagious form and who has not been treated releases the bacillus into the external environment, infecting other people. For this transmission to occur, there must be direct and prolonged contact with the untreated patient (BRASIL, 2010).

It is the causative agent of leprosy and has not yet been cultivated in vitro, making it a major challenge for microbiologists. In human tissues, they appear as straight or slightly curved bacilli between 2 and 8 mm long (OPROMOLLA, 2000).

In skin smears and histopathological sections, the bacilli are seen isolated, in varied groupings or in special arrangements called globia, peculiar to M. leprae, and result from the solid union of bacilli through a substance called glia (GOULART; PENNA; CUNHA, 2001).

The disease is transmitted mainly by living with patients of the virchowian or dimorphic type who have not yet been diagnosed and have not started treatment. These individuals have sufficient bacillary load to favour transmission. The main sources of bacteria are probably the mucous membranes of the upper airways. The Hansen's bacillus has the ability to infect a large number of individuals, but few fall ill. This property is not just a function of the intrinsic characteristics of the bacterium, but depends above all on its relationship with the host and the degree of endemicity of the environment (SANTOS; CASTRO; FALQUETO, 2008).

Leprosy is highly disabling because it causes nerve damage as a result of an inflammatory process in the peripheral nerves, the intensity, extent and distribution of which depend on the clinical form, the evolutionary phase of the disease and acute phenomena during reactional episodes. Neural damage causes changes in sensitivity, which in turn have consequences such as trauma and muscle weakness, generating physical deformities, which need to be diagnosed and treated early to prevent permanent disability and the emotional sequelae of infected individuals (LEITE et al., 2011).

The Ministry of Health defines a case of leprosy for treatment when one or more of the following criteria are present: skin lesion with altered sensitivity, nerve trunk thickening or positive skin smear microscopy. Treatment is based on specific chemotherapy, suppression of reactive outbreaks, prevention of physical disabilities along with physical and psychosocial rehabilitation (MELÃO et al., 2011).

In an endemic country like Brazil, the presence of a patch of skin with a different colour to the surrounding skin and with a change in sensitivity should be considered leprosy until proven otherwise. Sometimes leprosy initially presents itself differently, with intense reactive outbreaks. However, most of the time its diagnosis is not difficult and can be made by doctors and other health professionals, in the absence of the former. Let's remember that this country has more than five thousand municipalities and that our doctors are concentrated in just a few of them. Certainly, health professionals must be very well trained to carry out this diagnosis. In this regard, the Ministry of Health and the WHO have provided high-quality courses and educational materials to make this a reality (OPROMOLLA, BACCARELLI, 2003).

3.1 IMMUNOLOGY

Leprosy is influenced by the host's genetic factors, environmental factors such as nutritional status, BCG vaccination and the rate of exposure to M. leprae or other mycobacteria. The immune response is of fundamental importance for the body's defence against exposure to the bacillus. The alteration of the immune response is associated with the development of different clinical forms, in which the predominance of the cellular response is related to the milder clinical form of the disease (tuberculoid) and absence and the more severe clinical form (virchowian) (MENDONÇA et al, 2008).

Queiroz (2009) in an investigation carried out in endemic pockets of Indonesia revealed that more than half of the healthy population had antibodies against the mycobacterium, and around a quarter of them carried M. leprae-specific DNA molecules on the surface of their nasal mucosa.

The immune system is part of this important process which, when functionally healthy, becomes an efficient defence mechanism against foreign agents and neoplastic cells. For the immune system to fulfil its function, possible aggressors must be identified, i.e. only molecules foreign to the body's genetic code must be immunogenic (OPROMOLLA, 200).

The onset of the disease and its different clinical manifestations depend on the response of the individual's immune system to the bacillus, and can occur after a long incubation period, on average between two and seven years (BRASIL, 2010).

The main cellular components of the immune system are lymphocytes and antigen-presenting cells, represented mainly by langerhans cells, interdigitating cells, follicular dendritic cells and macrophages (OPROMOLLA, 2000).

The first line of interaction between M. leprae and humans is mediated by host cell receptors that recognise the molecular patterns of mycobacteria, the so-called pattern recognition receptors (PRRs). An example of this type of receptor, Toll-like receptors (TLRs) are essential for the recognition of pathogens by macrophages and dendritic cells during the innate immune response. Ten TLRs have already been identified, of which the heterodimers TLR2-TLR1, the homodimers TLR2 and TLR4 appear to be important for recognising mycobacteria (MENDONÇA et al, 2008).

3.2 LEPROSY NEUROPATHY

Peripheral neuropathy is the main cause of morbidity in leprosy and is responsible for the deformities and disabilities suffered by many people with the disease. Neural damage affects the fibres of the sensory, motor and autonomic peripheral nervous system. These nerve lesions are characterised by chronic or subacute infiltrates containing epithelioid cells or macrophages filled with bacilli. Nerve lesions are related to the individual's immune response, and limited studies indicate that the immunological mechanisms occurring in the nerves are similar to those already described in the skin (MENDONÇA et al, 2008).

In leprosy, autonomic, sensory and motor fibres are affected. Among the autonomic manifestations, the loss of sweating stands out, resulting in dry skin. Involvement of the cutaneous fibres results in loss of sensitivity to pain, cold and heat and, later on, also to touch. When the peripheral nerves are damaged, there is sensory, autonomic and motor involvement in the territory of the affected nerve(s). This results in loss of sensitivity (pain, cold, heat, touch, paresthesia and segmental position) and paresis, paralysis and muscle atrophy) (PROJETO DIRETIZES, 2003).

From the perspective of Opromolla and Baccarelli (2003), injuries to the peripheral nervous system can range from a simple localised impairment of a nerve fillet in the skin to the complete destruction of an important segment of the nerve trunk, such as the ulnar nerve in the elbow. More seriously, this impairment can occur before diagnosis, during treatment or even after treatment has ended.

Neural involvement is present in leprosy in any of its clinical forms, from the earliest forms of indeterminate leprosy, with cutaneous areas of thermal hypoanaesthesia, to the well-defined polar forms of the disease, such as the well-defined anaesthetic lesions of tuberculoid leprosy, through the dimorphic forms, to the "glove" and "boot" anaesthesia typical of advanced forms of lepromatous leprosy, with multiple affected nerve trunks. Neural involvement underlies all forms of leprosy (PIMENTEL et al, 2004).

3.3 CLINICAL MANIFESTATIONS

The incubation period for the disease is believed to be between 2 and 10 years. Skin lesions in leprosy can manifest as patches, plaques, skin infiltration, nodules, tubercles, alopecia, madarosis, trichiasis and mucosal lesions (RIDLEY and JOPLING,1966).

Other deformities can also originate from a secondary to severe infection due to trauma in non-sensitive areas, which can cause necrosis, which can often lead to amputation of the area, or osteomyelitis with a process of resorption of the bony extremities, particularly the fingers and toes (YAWALKAR, 2002).

Pure neural leprosy is usually diagnosed clinically by palpating the thickened nerve trunk, assessing skin sensitivity and muscle strength in the upper and lower limbs (YAWALKAR, 2002).

Brasil (2010) emphasises that leprosy manifests itself through skin lesions with decreased or absent sensitivity or numb lesions, due to the involvement of the peripheral cutaneous branches. The most common lesions are

- Whitish or reddish patches - change in skin colour, no relief.
- Papules - solid lesion with superficial, circumscribed elevation
- Infiltrations - Diffuse changes in the thickness of the skin.
- Tubercles - solid, raised lesion (external lumps).
- Nodules - solid lesions, more palpable than visible (internal lumps).

In the early stages of the disease, there may be increased sensitivity accompanied by a tingling sensation that can be mistaken for itching. Other general symptoms need to be appreciated:

- Oedema of hands and feet
- Fever and arthralgia
- Clogged, sore and dry nose
- Painful erythematous nodules
- General malaise
- Dry eyes

Considered a polymorphous disease, the expression of its clinical manifestations reflects the relationship between the host and the parasite. In individuals who fall ill, depending on the specific immunological response to the bacillus, the infection evolves in different ways. This immune response constitutes a spectrum that expresses the different clinical forms (LIMA et al, 2009).

The initial manifestation of the disease can be the indeterminate clinical form (I), where the host response is insufficiently differentiated to allow classification. It can evolve into a spontaneous cure or develop clinical aspects of the established disease within the spectrum, depending on its ability to mount a cellular immune response against M. leprae. The standard measure of cell-mediated immunity to the pathogen is the Mitsuda reaction, a delayed-type hypersensitivity reaction, which is assessed after an intradermal injection of dead bacilli applied to patients, whose endurance is measured after 3 to 4 weeks (GOULART; PENNA; CUNHA, 2001).

Sensitivity disorders resulting from the action of Mycobacterium leprae are characterised by the absence or reduction of thermal, painful and tactile sensitivities and can affect the skin, mucous membranes, peripheral nerves and, in extremely bacilliferous patients, the visual apparatus, causing deformities (ALVES et al, 2010).

Neural lesions can only be ramuscular, or in addition to the nerve fillets, superficial nerves and deeper nerve trunks can also be damaged. When the involvement is ramuscular, the alterations are essentially sensory and the first sensitivity to be altered is thermal, followed by painful and finally tactile sensitivity. After damaging the nerve branches, which are the first anatomical structures to be altered, the disease progresses proximally, affecting secondary branches and then the peripheral nerve trunks (SAMPAIO and RIVITTI, 2007).

3.4 DIAGNOSIS

Diagnosis is fundamental for identifying the case and treating it. Leprosy is an extremely complex disease, as it involves many organs and systems and has an important immunological component. However, in order to control a disease that is so widespread in our country, we need to see leprosy as a simple disease. In fact, its diagnosis is not complicated and requires very little equipment to be carried out with sufficient certainty (OPROMOLLA; BACCARELLI, 2003).

Skin smear microscopy (intradermal smear), whenever available, should be used as a complementary test to classify cases as paucibacillary (PB) or multibacillary (MB). Positive bacilloscopy classifies the case as MB, regardless of the number of lesions. It should be noted that a negative bacilloscopy result does not exclude the diagnosis of leprosy (BRASIL, 2010).

The baciloscopic examination has acquired greater importance after different authors showed that the recommendations of therapeutic regimens based solely on the number of lesions can lead to errors and cause relapse, bacillary persistence, therapeutic failure and/or insufficient treatment (PEDRO et al, 2010).

According to Brasil (2002), a clinical diagnosis is made through a physical examination, where a dermato-neurological assessment is carried out in an attempt to identify clinical signs of the disease. However, before starting the physical examination, an anamnesis should be taken, gathering information about the patient's clinical history, i.e. the presence of dermato-neurological signs and symptoms characteristic of the disease, and the epidemiological history, i.e. the source of infection.

The clinical diagnosis script consists of the following activities:

- Anamnesis - taking a clinical and epidemiological history;
- Dermatological assessment - identification of skin lesions with altered sensitivity
- Neurological assessment - identification of neuritis, disabilities and deformities.
- Diagnosis of reactional states
- Differential diagnosis
- Classification of the degree of physical disability.

Souza (1997) points out that the diagnosis of leprosy is based on some cardinal signs, such as the presence of anaesthesia in skin lesions, suggestive of the disease, the thickening of peripheral nerves, and the demonstration of M. leprae in lymph smears or histological tissue sections. For a correct diagnosis, it is necessary to understand the spectral concept of leprosy, which makes it possible to relate the evolving clinical course and the extent of cutaneous and neural involvement characteristic of each clinical form of the disease. Based on this knowledge, classifications are applied, which aid understanding and guide therapy.

Pedro et al (2010) emphasises that the result of the bacilloscopy contributes to the operational classification and consequently to the decision on the treatment regimen to be adopted. Cases diagnosed and treated as PB based solely on the number of lesions may receive insufficient treatment, resulting in a possible relapse.

3.5 CLASSIFICATION

For Opromolla (2000), classifying a disease is a way of understanding it better, and thus seeking a therapy that can control or even eradicate it. The more new facts that come to light as a result of his study, the more the classification changes and is completed.

The Ministry of Health recommends using the operational classification for leprosy, which considers PB to be cases with up to five lesions and clinically diagnosed as indeterminate and/or tuberculoid, and MB to be cases with more than five lesions and clinically classified as dimorphic and/or lepromatous. This strategy was adopted by the National Leprosy Control Programme (PNCH) in 2001 to define the therapeutic regimen and determine sovereignty during clinical examination (PEDRO et al, 2010).

In Brazil, the Madrid classification is adopted and the Ministry of Health suggests an operational classification with the following criteria: paucibacillary (PB) - cases with up to five skin lesions and/or only one nerve trunk affected and multibacillary (MB) - cases with more than five skin lesions and/or more than one nerve trunk affected. A positive bacilloscopy classifies the case as multibacillary, regardless of the number of lesions (ARAÚJO, 2003).

CHAPTER 4

THERAPEUTIC REGIMENS

According to data from the National Leprosy Service (1960), the most important legislative measures taken to control leprosy in the country up until the 20th century were: a law making it compulsory to isolate leprosy patients in Rio de Janeiro, enacted in 1756; the regulation signed in 1787 by D. Rodrigo Menezes for the hospital in Bahia; the issuing of appropriate legislation in 1883, which prohibited leprosy patients from working in certain professions. Rodrigo de Menezes in 1787 for the hospital in Bahia; the compulsory isolation of patients in the state of Pará in 1838; a ban on leprosy patients exercising certain professions in 1848 and, in 1883, the issuing of appropriate legislation with the creation of colony hospitals in Sabará (EIDT, 2004).

Polychemotherapy (MDT), which began in Brazil as a pilot project in some national Reference Centres, also began as a pilot project in the state of Mato Grosso in the municipality of Rondonópolis in 1987, later in the municipalities of Cuiabá and Cáceres. The need to expand the new therapeutic scheme triggered a new training process, considered essential for the new scheme to be implemented in the health services network. Training began in 1989, with the aim of both implementing the new therapeutic programme and increasing service coverage. For the period 1990-1994, the National Programme drew up the National Emergency Plan (PEM) and the state of Mato Grosso continued to increase staff training in order to comply with its State Plan. As a result of the training process, the coverage of control actions rose to 100% of municipalities in 1996, i.e. in every municipality there was at least one health unit with leprosy control actions (QUEIROZ, 2009).

By the end of the 1980s, most endemic countries had already implemented the polychemotherapy programme. Brazil started to do so in 1990 (BRASIL,1989), after having made great efforts to reorganise services in previous years as part of a national strategy to implement this therapeutic scheme, training large numbers of staff and investing in the equipment and supplies needed to set up a network of leprosy control services throughout the country (NOGUEIRA et al, 1995).

The implementation of MDT to control leprosy has marked a decrease in cases of the disease in Brazil in recent decades. However, the magnitude of the leprosy endemic remains an important health problem in the country. The emergence of resistance to specific drugs for its treatment, among other factors, is related to the occurrence of relapse (FERREIRA; IGNOTTI; GAMBA, 2011).

Opromolla and Baccarelli (2003) argue that MDT has had a very significant impact on leprosy control since its introduction. This association proved to be very effective in curing patients, reducing the fear of treatment and giving leprosy a new outlook - it became a curable disease. Perhaps this has been the most important factor, considering that the credibility of the cure of the disease is one of the most sensitive aspects for the community to come to see leprosy as a common disease - without fear or stigma.

PAUCIBACILLARY ADULTS: SIX-MONTH THERAPY

- Rifampicin® (RFM): monthly dose of 600 mg (2 capsules of 300 mg) with supervised administration.
- Dapsone® (DDS): monthly dose of 100 mg supervised and daily dose of 100 mg self-administered.
- Rifampicin® (RFM): monthly dose of 450 mg (1 capsule of 150 mg and 1 capsule of 300 mg) with supervised administration.

PAUCIBACILLARY INFANTS: SIX-MONTH THERAPY

Dapsone® (DDS): monthly dose of 50 mg supervised and daily dose of 50 mg self-administered.
Follow-up of cases: monthly visits for supervised dosing.

Discharge criteria: treatment will be completed with six (6) supervised doses within 9 months. At the 6ª dose, patients should undergo a dermatological examination, a simplified neurological assessment and a physical disability assessment, and be discharged as cured.

ADULT MULTIBACILLARY: 12-MONTH THERAPY

- Rifampicin® (RFM): monthly dose of 600 mg (2 capsules of 300 mg) with supervised administration.
- Dapsone® (DDS): monthly dose of 100 mg supervised and a daily dose of 100 mg self-administered.
- Clofazimine® (CFZ): monthly dose of 300 mg (3 capsules of 100mg) with supervised administration and a daily dose of 50 mg self-administered.

INFANT MULTIBACILLARY: 12-MONTH THERAPY

- Rifampicin® (RFM): monthly dose of 450 mg (1 capsule of 150 mg and 1 capsule of 300 mg) with supervised administration.
- Dapsone® (DDS): monthly dose of 50 mg supervised and a daily dose of 50 mg self-administered.

Clofazimine® (CFZ): monthly dose of 150 mg (3 capsules of 50 mg) with supervised administration and a dose of 50 mg self-administered every other day.

Follow-up of cases: monthly visits for supervised dosing.

- **Discharge criteria:** treatment will be completed with twelve (12) supervised doses within 18 months. At the 12ª dose, patients should undergo a dermatological examination, a simplified neurological assessment and a physical disability assessment, and be discharged as cured. MB patients who exceptionally do not show clinical improvement, with the presence of active lesions of the disease, at the end of the recommended treatment of 12 doses (cartridges) should be referred for assessment at a reference service (municipal, regional, state or national) to verify the most appropriate course of action for the case.

CHAPTER 5

REACTIONAL EPISODES

The Brazilian Leprosy Society (2003) and the Brazilian Dermatology Society (2003) define reactional episodes as acute phenomena superimposed on the chronic and insidious evolution of leprosy, potentially responsible for functional loss of peripheral nerves and aggravating disabilities. They result from the inflammatory process and immunological response, mediated by Mycobacterium leprae antigens, and are related to the bacillary load and the host's immune response.

Leprosy reactions reflect the phenomenon of acute hypersensitivity to Mycobacterium leprae antigens and are the result of an immunological process accompanied by an increase in pro-inflammatory cytokines, mainly IFN-y, IL-12, IL-1, IL-2, IL-4, IL-6, IL-8, IL-10, among others, as well as immune complexes. Reactions can occur before or, more often, during or after treatment. The duration and number of these outbreaks often depend on the clinical form, as well as the initial baciloscopic index (TEIXEIRA; SILVEIRA; FRANÇA, 2010).

According to Souza (2010), reaction episodes are type I or reverse reaction (indicating an increase in cellular immunity) and type II or erythema nodosum (exacerbation of humoral immunity). Type I reactions are characterised by erythema and oedema of pre-existing lesions and the appearance of new erythematous papules and plaques, most often in their vicinity. They occur in dimorphic clinical forms (tuberculoid-BT, dimorphic-BB, lepromatous-BL). There are apparently lepromatous cases, but they are actually very advanced dimorphs who, during treatment or even after it has been interrupted, exhibit reactional phenomena with lesions identical to those of the reactional dimorph.

Type II reactions or erythema nodosum occur in clinical lepromatous forms (LL), less frequently in the BL form. They are usually painful, erythematous papules or nodules, often preceded by fever, general malaise and painful adenopathy. The leprosy reaction is a major problem in the treatment of leprosy patients. In field practice, the burden of suffering produced by this morbidity is directly reflected in patients' lack of understanding of the reality that leprosy is curable (SOUZA, 2010).

CHAPTER 6

DISABILITY PREVENTION

Leprosy today represents a serious public health problem in Brazil, in addition to the aggravating factors inherent to any disease of socio-economic origin; the psychological repercussions generated by the physical disabilities resulting from the disease, when not properly treated, stand out. These disabilities are, in fact, the major cause of the patient's stigma and isolation in society. In order to avoid them, disability prevention (PI) actions include: health education, early diagnosis of the disease, regular MDT treatment and control of household contacts, including application of the BCG-ID vaccine; early detection and treatment of reactions and neuritis, support for maintaining the emotional condition and social integration (family, study, work, social groups) and guidance on self-care (VIEIRA et al, 2008).

Physical disability prevention and treatment activities should not be dissociated from MDT treatment. They will be developed during the follow-up of each case and should be integrated into the routine of the health unit's services, according to their degree of complexity. The adoption of disability prevention and treatment activities will be based on the information obtained from the neurological assessment at the time of leprosy diagnosis. This information refers to the neural impairment or physical disabilities identified, which deserve special attention in view of their consequences for the economic and social life of leprosy patients, or even their possible sequelae in those already cured (BRASIL, 2002).

There are numerous studies in the literature that identify the factors associated with the presence of physical disability at the time of diagnosis. Age, gender, schooling, clinical form, number of nerves affected and baciloscopic index are all factors associated with the presence of physical disability at the time of diagnosis. However, few studies have analysed these associations, checking the weight of each factor and the importance of this relationship. The variables associated with disability need to be better understood in order to plan and prioritise actions aimed at monitoring, treating and preventing disability in patients (MOSCHIONI, 2007).

During treatment with MDT, and in some cases after discharge, health professionals must be vigilant in relation to the disabling potential of the disease, in order to diagnose neuritis and reactions early and treat them appropriately, in order to prevent disabilities and prevent them from developing into deformities (BRASIL, 2002).

The long, asymptomatic incubation period of the disease and its insidious symptoms, coupled with the lack of technical training on the part of health professionals, can lead to diagnostic difficulties in the initial cases. The high percentage of patients with a degree of disability at the time of diagnosis reinforces the hypothesis that there is a large hidden prevalence which, in addition to the issue of deformities and stigmatisation of patients, influences the maintenance of the chain of transmission. The vast majority of leprosy patients do not have disabilities at the beginning of the disease, so the percentage of patients diagnosed with some degree of disability can be considered a late diagnosis, i.e. patients who were not detected at an early stage of the disease. Therefore, the risk of presenting deformities at the time of diagnosis increases significantly as the diagnosis is delayed (ALVES et al, 2010).

Eidt (2004) emphasises that multidrug therapy (polychemotherapy) makes M. leprae unviable, but does not recover or reverse the physical deformities that have already set in.

Alongside pharmacological treatment, measures to assess and prevent physical disabilities and health education activities, including self-care, should be developed.

JUSTIFICATIONS

Leprosy has always been present in human history. The magnitude of the disease, combined with its innate ability to generate conflicting feelings within the socio-economic-cultural environment, personifies and transcends historical eras.

It should be emphasised that over the years, especially after the advent of multidrug therapy and medical and laboratory advances, it has been possible to glimpse new perspectives with regard to early diagnosis and timely treatment.

Currently, the number of cases is changing according to the federal units analysed, showing differences in the percentage of prevalence and incidence.

Based on this emerging context, it is essential to carry out this research, which aims to characterise the previous and current behaviour of this disease in the state of Mato Grosso, highlighting profiles according to regional characteristics.

Notwithstanding these objectives, the results shown here could help the government to coordinate actions focused on prevention and health promotion.

CHAPTER 7

OBJECTIVES

5.1 General :

To analyse the geospatial behaviour of leprosy in the state of Mato Grosso (MT) between 2007 and 2011.

5.2 Specific(s):

To describe the profile of patients with MH in relation to the following variables: age, gender, colour/race, schooling, marital status, place of residence.

Classifying the epidemiological profile of leprosy according to socio-demographic information.

To describe the spatial distribution of MH cases in the state of Mato Grosso according to place of residence.

Calculate prevalence rates for the period, based on place of residence.

To verify associations between socio-economic and demographic indicators in the geographical area.

To demonstrate the prevalence indicators of leprosy in children under fifteen in the state of Mato Grosso.

Relating vulnerability factors to leprosy morbidity indicators

CHAPTER 8

CASUISTRY AND METHOD

5.3 TYPE OF STUDY

This is an ecological, descriptive, cross-sectional study with secondary data from 2007 to 2011, using spatial data analysis techniques to analyse Hansen's disease cases in the state of Mato Grosso (MT).

5.4 STUDY SITE

Mato Grosso, a Brazilian state whose capital is Cuiabá, has an estimated population of 3,035,122 inhabitants, spread over an area of 903,366.192 km and with a population density of 3.36 (inhab/km^2). In terms of its geographical division, the state is made up of 141 municipalities (Figure 2) (IBGE, 2010).

It is the country's third largest state in terms of area and lies to the west of the Centre-West region. Most of its territory is occupied by the Legal Amazon. Its borders are Amazonas and Pará to the north; Tocantins and Goiás to the east; Mato Grosso do Sul to the south; Rondônia and Bolivia to the west. The state of Mato Grosso has a time zone of four hours less than world time GMT and its predominant climate is the tropical super-humid monsoon. Its economy is based on agriculture, livestock farming, mining and industry. Mato Grosso is one of Brazil's main soya producers and exporters (SÓ GEOGRAFIA, 2013).

The state can be defined as a mosaic of natural riches represented by forests, savannahs, savannahs and wetlands. In the south-central region the cerrado predominates, in the north the Amazon rainforest and in the southeast the pantanal. Mato Grosso's privileged and strategic geographical location should also be highlighted, as it is an important trading post, linking corridors that connect the Atlantic to the Pacific. Today, Mato Grosso's road links to the Pacific ports of Chile and Peru, via Bolivia, are a reality (GOVERNMENT OF THE STATE OF MATO GROSSO, 2013).

Betting on tourism as one of the most important economic activities in the age of globalisation, generating wealth and jobs, the government has invested in structuring the sector, training specialised staff to serve tourists well through the "Quality Brigades" programme, improving transport and communication infrastructure and seeking to attract private investment in the hotel sector (GOVERNMENT OF THE STATE OF MATO GROSSO, 2013).

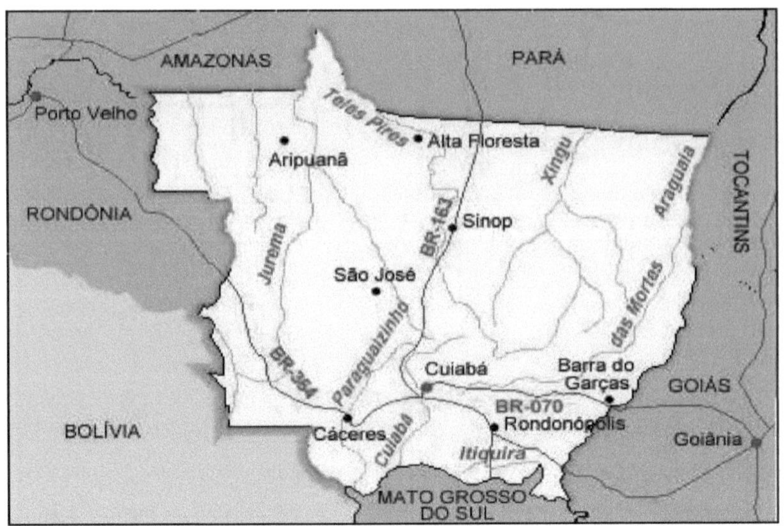

Figure 2 - Spatial location of the state of Mato Grosso.
Source: www.sogeografia.com.br/Conteudos/GeografiaFisica/Cartografia

8.3 DATA SOURCES

8.3.1 DATABASES FOR REGISTERED CASES OF MH

The data was obtained from the Unified Health System database (DATASUS) and TABNET. In conjunction, the Notifiable Diseases Information System (SINAN) was another tool used in the study. The age groups of the entire population were extracted, keeping the focus of the analyses on those under fifteen years of age. Since leprosy is a compulsorily notifiable disease, all diagnosed patients must be notified by health professionals.

In this way, it was possible to obtain reliable information about the desired sample. The place of work was the municipality's Epidemiological Surveillance Department, attached to the Municipal Health Secretariat.

8.3.2 STUDY VARIABLES

To establish the desired morbidity, the variables used to draw up the clusters were: demographic and socio-economic indicators, operational classification, new cases in children under fifteen, general detection coefficient and degree of disability at diagnosis.

8.4 DATA ANALYSIS PROCEDURE

For the first stage, the data was collected, organised and summarised in an Excel® spreadsheet and then analysed descriptively using absolute numbers, percentages and proportions.

In the second stage, the spatial distribution of leprosy cases in the state of Mato Grosso, Brazil was analysed using the GEODA software (ANSELIN, 2005), version 0.9.5, Spatial Analysis Laboratory, University of Illinois at Urbana- Champaign, Urbana, United States. As with the descriptive analysis, a 5% significance level was used for the spatial statistical analysis.

To calculate the spatial autocorrelation rates for morbidity, socioeconomic factors and demographic indicators for each city, the Global Moran's Index (I) was used for uni- and bivariate analysis (ANDRADE, 2009). This index measures both spatial autocorrelation and the weighted neighbourhood matrix, indicating that the rates in a given region may be similar to those in neighbouring regions. Moran's values can vary between -1 and +1. According to (PEROBELLI and HADDAD, 2006) values greater or less than the expected value of Moran's I [E (I) = -1 / (N - 1)] indicate positive or negative autocorrelation, respectively.

Moran I values between 0 and 1 indicate a positive (direct) spatial association. This indicates that regions with high values for the variable are surrounded by regions that also have high variable values (ANDRADE, 2009). Similarly, regions with low variable values are surrounded by regions with low variable values. Negative Moran's I values (from 0 to -1) represent negative (inverse) spatial association. Therefore, regions with high values are surrounded by regions with low variable values, while regions with low Moran's I values are surrounded by neighbours with high variable values (ANDRADE, 2009).

Once the spatial weight matrix had been selected, which for this study is the Queen, the presence of spatial dependence was checked using the Global and Local Spatial Autocorrelation measures. Global Spatial Autocorrelation is used to check the randomness or autocorrelation of the data, whether the values in a given region are similar to those in other neighbouring regions (ANDRADE, 2009).

Spatial Empirical Bayes (SANTOS; RODRIGUES; LOPES, 2005) was used to smooth the rates relating to population size. The methodology estimates corrected rates from the observed values using Bayesian inference concepts. The global empirical Bayes estimator calculates a weighted average between the gross rate for the locality and the global rate for the region (ratio between the total number of cases and the total population).

The local empirical Bayes estimator includes spatial effects, calculating the estimate locally using only the geographical neighbours of the area in which the rate is to be estimated, converging towards a local average rather than a global average. Corrected rates are less unstable, as they take into account not only the area's information, but also the information from its neighbourhood. Maps based on these estimates are more interpretative and informative (SANTOS; RODRIGUES; LOPES, 2005).

According to Almeida (2004), Moran's I is a measure of global association, which can be univariate, o or bivariate and may or may not conform to local patterns, and can hide local patterns of association.

Univariate Moran's analysis was carried out to check for global spatial autocorrelation (AMARAL, 2010). Univariate analysis is the examination of the distribution of cases of just one variable at a time. The most basic format for presenting univariate data is to report all the individual cases, listing the attribute (category) of each case studied in the variable in question. Instead of presenting the list with all the data, you can distribute the data in frequency tables without losing any detail. We can present frequency distributions of grouped data (marginal data) (AMARAL, 2010).

Bivariate analysis was used to make the association between morbidity rates and socioeconomic variables (VIEIRA; REMACRE, 2001). In bivariate regression analysis, the correlation coefficient is often used to judge the relationship between two variables, and assumptions are also made about the linearity of the data in order to make spatial and temporal interpretations, etc.

For a greater level of detail, we used the LISA (Local Indicators of Spatial Association) spatial statistic and Moran's scatter plots, which make it possible to observe the existence of spatial clusters, places with high or low values and the regions that most contribute to the existence of spatial autocorrelation (ANDRADE, 2009).

Local **Spatial Autocorrelation -** *Local Indicator of Spatial Association (LISA)* is a statistic that aims to identify significant spatial association patterns for each area analysed. Its values are proportional to the values of the global spatial association indicators (ANDRADE, 2009).

CHAPTER 9

RESULTS and DISCUSSION

Based on data from DATASUS/TABNET/SINAN, between 2007 and 2011, the state of Mato Grosso registered a total of 13,648 cases of leprosy, with a reduction in the number of patients over the period analysed (table 3). The economically active 40 to 69 age group accounted for 6583 notifications, closely followed by the 15 to 39 age group, with 5,386 cases (graph 4) (BRASIL, 2008). In its epidemiological study, it showed that the coefficient rate averaged 60.77/100,000 inhabitants. Considering that this condition can lead to serious functional damage to patients, this brings to light a major public health problem. It should also be noted that patients with motor, sensory and autonomic damage often have to take time off work, resulting in a loss of productive and financial strength for the worker and for the country (GOVERNO DO CEARÁ, 2013) reveals that leprosy affects the economically active population aged between 20 and 59, with 63.1% in the phase of the individual's greatest productivity, having social and economic repercussions on the lives of those affected by the disease.

Romão and Mazzoni (2013) report that with regard to the distribution of leprosy by age group, in relation to the absolute frequency of cases, it was observed that 121 cases or (42.9%) of the total diagnoses in the period were included in the 20 to 39 age group. This was followed by the 40 to 59 age group, with 95 cases or (33.68%) of the records. The lowest number of diagnoses was in the 5 to 9 year-old age group, with 2 (0.70%) cases.

According to (BRASIL ESCOLA) it is the second most populous state in the Centre-West region, with only the state of Goiás having a larger population (6,003,788 inhabitants). The majority of Mato Grosso residents live in urban areas (82 per cent), while the rural population comprises 18 per cent. In recent years, Mato Grosso has received considerable migratory flows as a result of the expansion of the agricultural frontier. The state's population is made up of people from different ethnic backgrounds (BRASIL ESCOLA).

According to the latest ministerial bulletins, leprosy incidence and prevalence rates are falling in all federal units. In Mato Grosso, the incidence rate showed a reduction over the period studied (Graph 3). Nevertheless, the data presented still keeps the state of Mato Grosso at the top of the total number of cases in Brazil (BRASIL, 2012). The priority municipalities are located in all units of the Federation, but are mainly concentrated in the states of Maranhão, Mato Grosso, Pará and Rondônia. The metropolitan regions of Recife and Fortaleza are also considered to be of great epidemiological importance.

Despite the significant reduction in the leprosy prevalence coefficient in Brazil, some regions require intensified action to eliminate the disease, justified by a pattern of high endemicity (BRASIL, 2012).

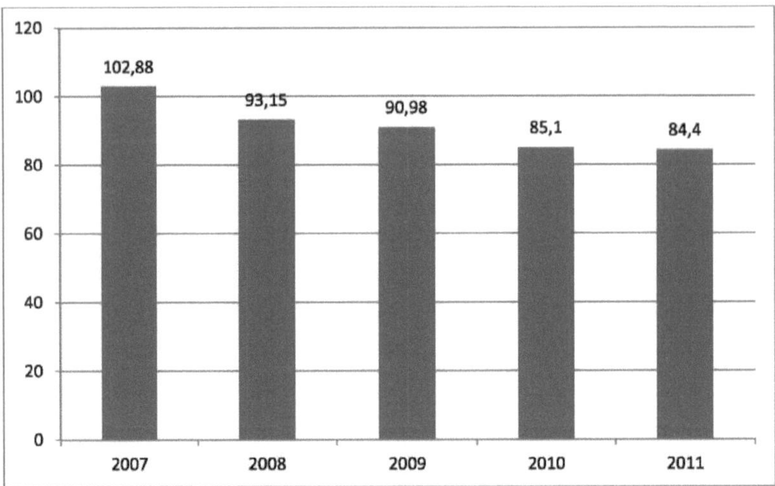

Graph 3: Time series of the incidence rate in relation to the total number of leprosy cases in the population between 2007 and 2011.
Source: DATASUS/TABNET/SINAN

High incidence data reveal a progressive behaviour of the pathology within the geographical limits of the state. This reduction visualised above is still below expectations (SOUZA, 2012), who argues that epidemiological control of a communicable disease is defined as reducing the disease burden to a locally acceptable level.

Brasil (2008) states that the detection coefficient of new cases is a function of the actual incidence and the diagnostic agility of health services, and the relationship between detection and actual incidence comprises the hidden prevalence, which is directly linked to the transmission of the disease. Reducing leprosy transmission presupposes reducing the hidden prevalence through agile detection, which reduces the time of illness before diagnosis.

Of Brazil's five macro-regions, four have a high prevalence: North (4.54/1,000); Centre-West (3.41/1,000); South-East (1.72/1,000); South (1.24/1,000). The North-East has a medium prevalence (0.86/1,000), but this lower rate is not due to a lower number of patients, but to low notification (QUEIROZ; PUNTEL, 1997).

At the state level, the crude detection rate is four times higher in MT. The differences in detection rates between the states are more significant in the under-15 age group (SOUZA, 2012). The distribution of the number of cases of the disease is dissimilar between geographical areas, making it necessary to know the local epidemiological situation in order to define priority actions according to each situation (SOBRINHO, 2007).

From 1996 to 1999, the highest leprosy detection rates were concentrated in six regions: São Félix do Araguaia, Água Boa, Barra do Garças, Diamantino, Tangará da Serra and Cáceres, located in the Centre-North, Southwest and Northeast regions of the state, all with detection coefficients between 13.99 and 20.99/10. 000 inhabitants.During this period, there were five regional centres (Sinop, Colíder, Alta Floresta, Juína and Juara), located in the north of the state, which had lower detection rates, one of them below the hyperendemic level (<4/10,000) (QUEIROZ, 2009).

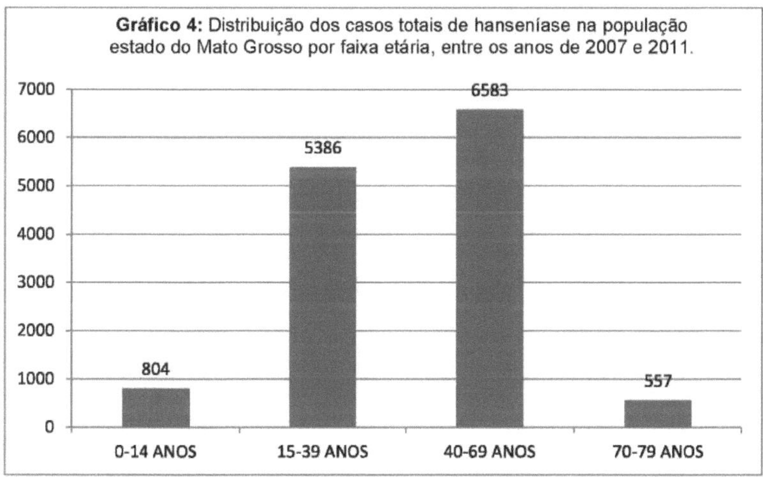

Queiroz (2009) observed that the coefficients are higher in the older age groups, especially in the 15 to 44 and 45 and over age groups, with an increase in these two age groups in the intermediate period and a reduction in the last period, considered an indicator of the trend of the leprosy endemic.

Paes et al (2001) described that with regard to age, there was a predominance of young adults aged between 15 and 30 (32.3%) and this percentage increases if we take into account the population up to 60 years of age, which is worrying from a socio-economic point of view, due to the disabilities that the disease causes and these individuals being in the productive phase of life.

In Brazil, leprosy affects more than 500,000 people, most of them of working age, negatively influencing their work, family formation and social integration (SIMÕES; DELELLO, 2005).

Within the under-15 age group, the 10-14 age group predominated, with 503 cases. (ALENCAR, 2008) reports that the country has an average detection rate in children under 15 of 0.53 new cases per 10,000 inhabitants (absolute number 2,980 new cases), which is considered very high. In the last five years, the average number of new cases detected in this population in Brazil has been 4,000.

Souza (2012) emphasises that the population of MT exceeds that of MS by almost half a million inhabitants, but with narrow differences in the proportion between the sexes and age groups. Municipalities with a higher proportion of young people under the age of 15 were identified in MT.

Mato Grosso has worrying rates in children under fifteen, which place it at the centre of the Ministry of Health's actions. (BRASIL, 2008) points out that once again the commitment of the Legal Amazon in relation to leprosy is evident, with the state of Tocantins occupying the first position in the country, with a coefficient of 23.6/100.000 inhabitants, Mato Grosso in second place with a coefficient of 19.74/100,000, Pará in third place with 18.07/100,000, Maranhão in fourth place with 16.80/100,000, Rondônia in fifth place with 14.16/100,000, Acre in seventh place with 12.10/100,000 and Roraima in eighth place with a coefficient of 11.27/100,000 inhabitants. Considering the number of occurrences in the nine states of the region, the Legal Amazon concentrated 46.4 per cent of new cases in children under 15 registered in the country in 2007.

Barbieri and Marques (2009) corroborate this by saying that leprosy can affect all age groups, but is more common in adults. The prevalence of the disease in children and adolescents under the age of 15 is higher in endemic countries, revealing the persistence of bacillus transmission and the difficulties health programmes face in controlling the disease.

The epidemiology of leprosy in children under fifteen in the state of Mato Grosso reflects an important condition, emphasising that this disease can generate a series of relevant functional, social and psychological changes in these adolescents (PONTE; NETO, 2005) understands that an adolescent who is in a phase of change and adaptation to leprosy can interfere with the construction of their life, due to the changes that, depending on the case, they will have to go through; there may even be school dropouts, an increase in crises, depreciation of self-image, with consequent alteration of self-esteem.

Since leprosy is a stigmatising disease that causes physical and psychological disorders, and taking into account that in adolescence people are building their adult identity and are therefore more vulnerable, this reality led us to be interested in researching this subject, arising from the need to know if the characteristics of this disease affect the establishment of this new identity (PONTE; NETO, 2005).

With regard to demographic socio-economic indicators, the state of Mato Grosso had an average Gini Index of 0.55 and an illiteracy rate of 11.8 (IBGE, 2010), considering the years 1991, 2000 and 2010.

The most widely used indicator to measure income inequality is the Gini index, which ranges from zero to one. A Gini index close to one means that income is highly concentrated in the hands of a small minority; on the other hand, a Gini index close to zero represents a more egalitarian distribution. By this indicator, Brazil is one of the most unequal countries in the world, with a Gini of around 0.5605. To give you an idea, most developed countries have a Gini between 0.25 and 0.40. In Mato Grosso, the index is around 0.5284. The state with the lowest inequality (and poverty rate) in Brazil is Santa Catarina, which has a Gini of 0.4630 (DIÁRIO DE CUIABÁ, 2009).

Portal Mato Grosso (2013) reports that the illiteracy rate in the Northeast, historically recognised as having the highest number of illiterate people in the country, fell from 22.4% (2004) to 18.7% (2009). The information was released today (8) by the Brazilian Institute of Geography and Statistics (IBGE), which recorded a nationwide reduction in the number of people who could not read or write in 2009. The reduction, considered by the IBGE itself to be "slight", produced an illiteracy rate of 9.7 per cent last year, with just over 14 million people registered in this condition throughout the country. According to the National Household Sample Survey (PNAD 2009), the drop in the rate differed between the major regions, with the South and Southeast showing the lowest levels of illiteracy. In 2004, the illiteracy rate was 11.5 per cent. The survey also revealed that the rate increases with age. "The highest concentration of illiterates was registered among people belonging to the highest age groups: 92.6 per cent of them were aged 25 or over." (PORTAL MATO GROSSO, 2013).

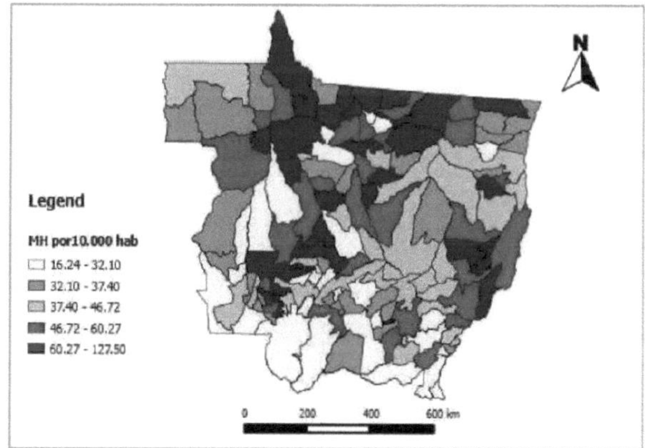

Figure 3 - SPACE DISTRIBUTION OF HANSENIASIS IN THE POPULATION OF THE STATE OF MATO GROSSO. INCIDENCE RATE PER 10,000 INHABITANTS

The geospatial analysis of the first map shows that the state of Mato Grosso has areas with rates above those recommended by the Ministry of Health, the World Health Organisation and the Pan American Health Organisation, which is less than 1 case per 10,000 inhabitants. 27 municipalities had rates ranging from 60.27 to 127.50 per 10,000 inhabitants. Brasil (2013) corroborates this condition, pointing out that the spatial pattern of leprosy remains the same, with prevalence rates predominating in municipalities located on the edge of the Amazon, Maranhão, Mato Grosso, Pará and Tocantins, and in some metropolitan areas of the Northeast.

28 municipalities had rates of between 46.72 and 60.27 per 10,000 inhabitants. It is imperative to emphasise that the state of Mato Grosso shares a border with the aforementioned states, potentialising a migratory influx of a population contingent into the state's 141 municipalities. Considering the intrinsic characteristics of the spread of leprosy, such as agglomerations and

prolonged inter-human contact. These socio-demographic characteristics may justify this spatial condition.

Residences and neighbouring municipalities where a leprosy patient has been diagnosed are the main risk areas for new cases of the disease, corroborating the need to examine contacts as extremely important for controlling the endemic.

The state of Mato Grosso has an essentially agricultural economy and growing urbanisation, but it still has extensive areas of woodland and forest. The existence of these extensive "unoccupied" areas has been a strong attraction for migrants, fuelling rapid economic growth in recent years. The migratory process alters the epidemiological structure of the areas where migrants leave as well as those where they arrive, with immediate repercussions on the individual and collective risks of disease. The relationship between man and the environment includes the action of nature on man and human action modelling nature. (MAGALHÃES et al 2011)

According to Souza (2012), migration is cited as a factor that can artificially increase or decrease the prevalence of leprosy in some areas or introduce patients to unaffected areas. However, the sporadic introduction of imported leprosy cases has not produced secondary cases in non-endemic countries.

Magalhães et al (2011) point out that the geographical presentation in foci, without a definitive explanation, the prolonged subclinical evolution of the disease, associated with the intense migratory movements of recent decades and the concentration of the population in cities make the geography of leprosy one of the most difficult chapters in global, regional and local nosogeography.

Brasil (2011) emphasises that the state of Pará still has areas with active transmission regions, with high detection in children under fifteen. However, the highest levels of the endemic are found in the North, Centre-West and Northeast regions, which together account for 53.5% of reported cases.

Although trend studies show that the leprosy endemic is decreasing, geoprocessing of new cases shows that there are hotspots of recent transmission, particularly in the nine states of the legal Amazon (BRASIL, 2011).

In Brazil, the states with the highest detections and the most unfavourable evolution of the endemic have historically been located in the North and Centre-West regions, which shows an uneven regional evolution, suggesting the existence of geographical contexts with different vulnerabilities to the social production of leprosy. Data from 2007 from the Ministry of Health shows the commitment of the Legal Amazon in relation to leprosy, since this area, which has 12.9% of Brazil's population, concentrates 38.9% of the new cases detected in the country (MAGALHÃES et al 2011).

As a priority indicator for monitoring the progression of leprosy in federal units, the prevalence rate in Mato Grosso has remained high (5 - 9.99/ 10,000 inhabitants), placing the state in an unfavourable position. Between 2003 and 2012, there was a drop in the state's overall detection rate, which ended at 80.34 per 100,000 inhabitants, the highest in Brazil (BRASIL, 2013).

Considering the current international pacts for the elimination of leprosy as a global public health problem, there are possibilities regarding the quantitative persistence of the number of leprosy cases in the state. Although the last ten years have seen a statistical drop in incidence, we are still a long way from achieving the Millennium Development Goals 20112015. (BRASIL, 2013)

Brasil (2008) presents the evolution of the detection coefficients of new cases in the total population and according to sex. It can be seen that the average coefficients between 2001 and 2007 were 8.94/100,000 inhabitants for males and 22.63/100,000 for females. The values for males ranged from 23.64/100,000 in 2007 to 32.02/100,000 in 2003, and for females from 17.78/100,000 in 2001 to 25.59/100,000 in 2003. The evolution of this indicator over the monitored period showed higher figures for males than for females over the seven years observed, in proportions ranging from 20.1 per cent in 2003 to 24.8 per cent in 2007.

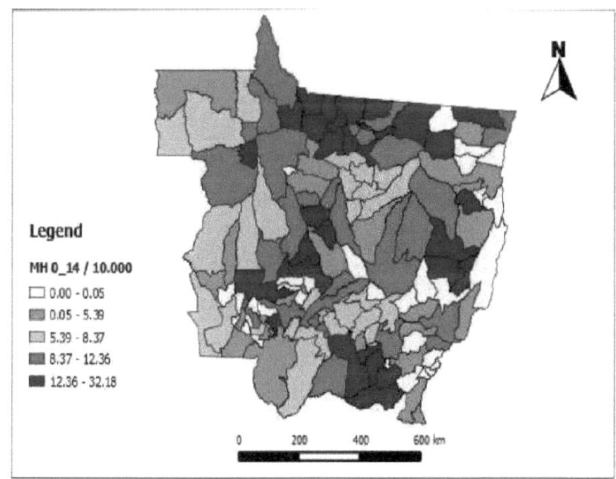

Figure 4 - GEOESPACE DISTRIBUTION OF HANSENIASIS CASES IN UNDER-14S. ADJUSTED RATE PER 10,000 INHABITANTS

By analysing the geospatial distribution of the second map, which deals with the number of leprosy cases in children under 15 per 10,000 inhabitants, we can see that there is an epidemiological connection with the first figure, where it is possible to establish the endemic condition of this pathology in the youngest forms.

Reducing cases in children under 15 is a priority for the PNCH. These cases are related to recent disease and active transmission foci, and their epidemiological monitoring is relevant to leprosy control. The target set by the PNCH for the PAC is to reduce the detection rate of new cases in children under 15 by 10.0 per cent in the country by 2011. The evolution of the detection coefficients of new cases in the total population and in children under 15, in the period from 1994 to 2007

(BRASIL, 2008)

The detection rate of new cases in children under 15 is related to the level of endemicity and reflects early exposure to M. leprae. For 2002, this rate in Brazil was 0.70 per 10,000 inhabitants, with wide variations by region, ranging from 0.30/10,000 inhabitants in the South to 2.23/10,000 inhabitants in the North. In Mato Grosso, records indicate a detection rate of 2.84/10,000 inhabitants in children under 15, which places the state in the hyperendemic parameter (QUEIROZ, 2009).

In their studies, Vieira et al (2008) report that in endemic countries, the child population comes into contact with bacilliferous patients at an early age, which contributes to the detection of the disease in children aged between three and five, with cases rarely being seen in children under two, especially of the lepromatous form. These data demonstrate the risk of children under 15 becoming ill with leprosy in endemic countries.

The detection coefficients of new cases in children under 15 years of age, distributed by state, for 2007, are presented. Once again, the commitment of the Legal Amazon in relation to leprosy is evident, with the state of Tocantins occupying the first position in the country, with a coefficient of 23.6/100,000 inhabitants, Mato Grosso occupying the second position, with a coefficient of 19.74/100.000, Pará third with 18.07/100,000, Maranhão fourth with 16.80/100,000, Rondônia fifth with 14.16/100,000, Acre seventh with 12.10/100,000 and Roraima eighth with 11.27/100,000 inhabitants. Considering the number of occurrences in the nine states of the region, the Legal Amazon concentrated 46.4 per cent of new cases in children under 15 registered in the country in 2007 (BRASIL, 2008).

As one of the Ministry's main indicators, this data prompts discussions about the progression of leprosy at a state level. Considering the pathophysiology and incubation period of the disease, this data shows an active circulation of this mycobacterium in our population. According to Ferreira and Alvarez (2001), although leprosy is considered to be a disease of adults and young adults, there are numerous reports of cases of this disease in age groups under fifteen. The reason for this is that there is an increase in the chain of transmission of the bacillus in the community, as well as a deficiency in the surveillance and control of the disease. In endemic countries, the child population comes into contact with bacilliferous patients at an early age, and it is possible to observe a detection of the disease among children aged between three and five years old, and cases are rarely observed in children under two years old, especially of the virchowian form.

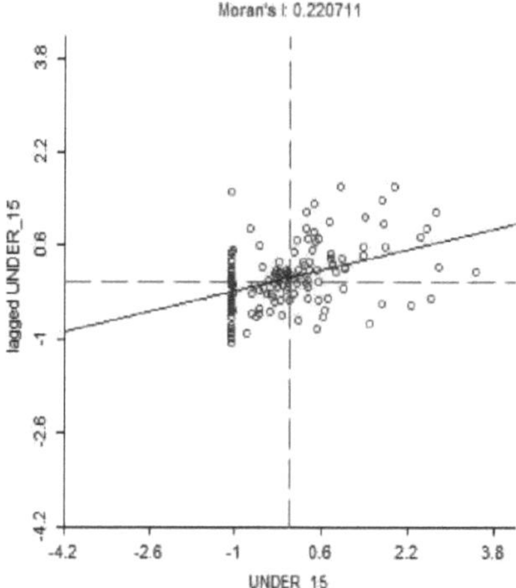

Graph 5 - MORAN I DISPERSION DIAGRAM FOR INCIDENCE RATES IN UNDER-15S IN THE PERIOD 2007-2001.

The univariate analysis of morbidity rates from MH in children under 15 indicated the existence of a positive spatial autocorrelation (I = 0.220711, p = 0.001). This shows that cities with high morbidity rates from MH in children under 15 tend to be surrounded by neighbouring cities with similar high morbidity rates from MH.

The occurrence of leprosy in children can be considered an indicator of the prevalence of the disease in the general population and its detection is important for determining the level of transmission. Leprosy is considered an adult disease due to its long incubation period, but children are also susceptible to it. Therefore, in endemic areas and when there are cases in the family, the risk of children becoming ill increases (IMBIRIBA et al, 2005).

Moran's scatter diagram according to the spatial weight matrix showed a positive auto-correlation with the population of children under fifteen exposed to the disease within the boundaries of the municipalities with a high number of cases. This positive distribution shows that municipalities with a high number of leprosy cases are surrounded by other areas with high incidence rates. These geographically close areas allowed the formation of some epidemiological clusters, in order to visualise the regions with the greatest influx of cases.

These data are in line with ministerial statistics and the literature, reinforcing the endemic nature of Mato Grosso in terms of prevalence and detection rates, suggesting early contact of the younger population with the bacillus. This is in line with (IMBIRIBA et al, 2005), which reports that the continued high levels of leprosy endemicity suggest that children may be contacts of cases not yet detected by the health system. In conditions of high transmissibility and early exposure to the bacillus, the likelihood of becoming ill increases and so detection in this age group is taken as an indicator of the greater severity of the endemic. In order to contribute to actions to control the disease, the aim of this study was to analyse the epidemiological situation of leprosy in children in urban areas.

Childhood leprosy is a public health problem, reflecting early exposure, community transmission and the limited effectiveness of control programmes. Several studies indicate a high risk of leprosy among household contacts, especially those living with multibacillary (MB) cases. The importance of studying leprosy in childhood stems initially from the fact that this disease affects the skin, the largest and most visible organ of the body, and the risk of physical disfigurement. The under-18 age group represents 36 per cent of the Brazilian population. The majority of leprosy cases in this age group are non-contagious, with few skin lesions and negative bacilloscopy. If diagnosis and treatment are timely and correct, the tendency is for a cure without sequelae (FERREIRA; ANTUNES, 2008).

Alencar et al (2008) in their study in the municipality of Fortaleza on the prevalence of leprosy in children under the age of 15 observed a high proportion of case detection in children over the last 13 years.

Considering the possibility of underreporting of cases, including in this specific population, the scale of the disease in the municipality increases even more.

In their study, Alencar and Lana (2008) showed that the percentage of cases in children under fifteen is striking. This result justifies the adoption of more specific prevention and control measures aimed at this group of the population, such as active searches in schools and nurseries, lectures explaining the signs and symptoms of the disease and intensified examinations of communicants. The need for careful population surveys at this age is emphasised, both for detecting cases and for better follow-up in endemic areas.

The high endemicity of the disease in an area will lead to multiple exposures of the population to the bacillus, in addition to the fact that these exposures occur in the first few years of life. Thus, one of the most sensitive indicators in relation to the leprosy control situation is the percentage of cases in young people. The occurrence of leprosy in children under 15 years of age indicates the precocity of exposure and the persistence of transmission of the disease, making it an important element in assessing its magnitude. In 2005, Brazil had a leprosy detection coefficient in children under 15 of 0.6 per 10,000 inhabitants, a rate considered high by Ministry of Health (MoH) standards. In the same year, the detection coefficient in the Southeast region was 0.2 cases/10,000 inhabitants and in the state of Minas Gerais, detection in children represented 5.95 per cent of the total number of new cases, which corresponds to 0.3 cases/10,000 inhabitants (LANA et al, 2007).

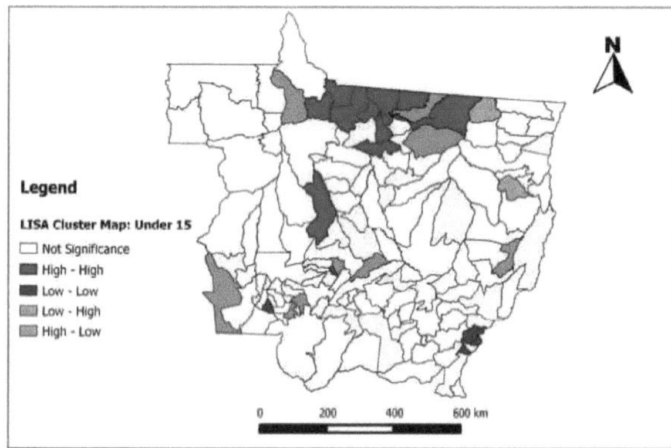

Figure 5 - AGGREGATION OF EPIDEMIOLOGICAL CLUSTERS FOR THE SPACE DISTRIBUTION OF HANSENIASIS CASES IN THE PERIOD 2007 TO 2011.

The univariate LISA analysis made it possible to detect clusters based on the similarities between the cities (Map 4). We can therefore classify these groups of cities using the following categories: (1) high-high, i.e. cities with high MH morbidity with surrounding neighbours also with high MH morbidity, (2) low-low, i.e. cities with low MH indices with neighbours with low MH indices, (3) low-high, i.e. cities with low MH indices with neighbours with high MH morbidity, and (4) highlow, i.e. cities with high MH morbidity with neighbours with indices (Map 4). Six high-high clusters were identified involving 10 cities, which are located in the northern region of the state on the border with the state of Amazonas.

The DATASUS data guided the identification of clusters to monitor the behaviour of leprosy in Brazil. The clusters define areas with the highest risk and where the majority of cases are found. Detecting the areas most at risk of the disease allows the control programme to be directed towards areas where transmission is greatest, with a focus on geographically continuous areas and greater epidemiological effectiveness. The cluster approach avoids ignoring silent areas due to a low detection effort or prioritising municipalities with many cases due to the size of their population rather than their greater risk. (BRASIL, 2008)

However, while there is no doubt about the existence of a cluster in a given area, its precise delimitation is not so clear and there is a need for an analysis that includes more precise local information and the knowledge generated by the physical proximity of the facts and the concrete experience of leprosy control in order to better delimit these higher risk areas. The cases were spatially allocated according to the geographical coordinates of the municipalities' headquarters in order to approximate their real location.

The local association indicator (LISA) was used to establish clusters based on the results of the maps and the Moran I diagram. Using GEODA's LISA MAP tool, it was possible to identify significant clusters (p <5%) in areas with high incidence rates, surrounded by municipalities with high numbers of cases.

The spatial analysis of the distribution of leprosy in the municipality of Duque de Caxias identified a cluster in the south-northwest, which was not directly related to campaign actions or decentralisation. This finding reinforces the possibility of this type of analysis being used as an important tool for identifying critical areas of the endemic and for assessing the impact of strategic actions to combat the disease carried out in the region, including risk factors related to the social, economic and health conditions of exposed individuals (DUARTE- CUNHA et al, 2012).

It is interesting to consider these clusters in relation to the state's geodemographic conditions. Souza (2012) stresses that the hyperendemicity of leprosy currently found in the agricultural frontier area, which contiguously covers several states in the Centre-West, North and North-East regions of Brazil, suggests that there is a relationship between the endemic process of leprosy and the occupation of new places; where the demographic movement necessary to clear a virgin field of mechanisation seems to encourage the incidence of the disease.

Graph 6 - MORN DISPERSION DIAGRAM, ACCORDING TO THE SPACE MATRIX FOR THE INCOME VARIABLE, IN THE PERIOD 2007-2001.

A)

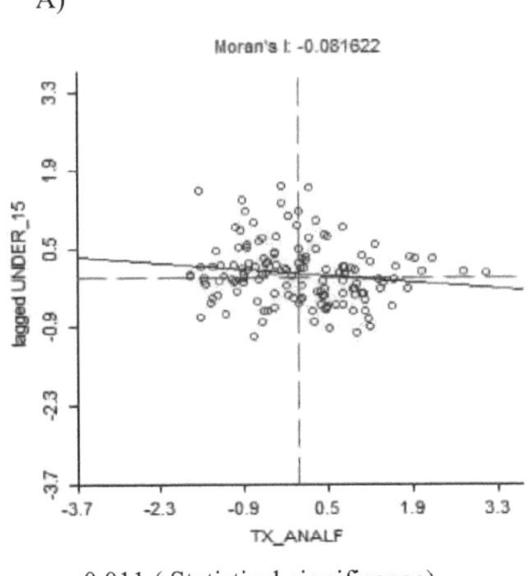

p = 0.011 (Statistical significance)

B)

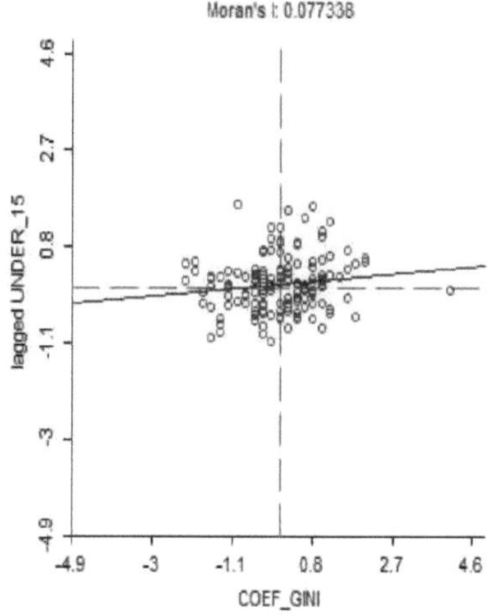

p − 0.020 (Statistical significancc)

C)

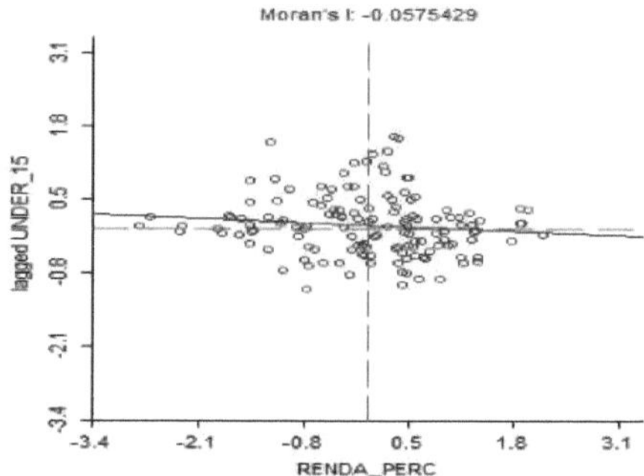

p = 0.063 (Not significant)

D)

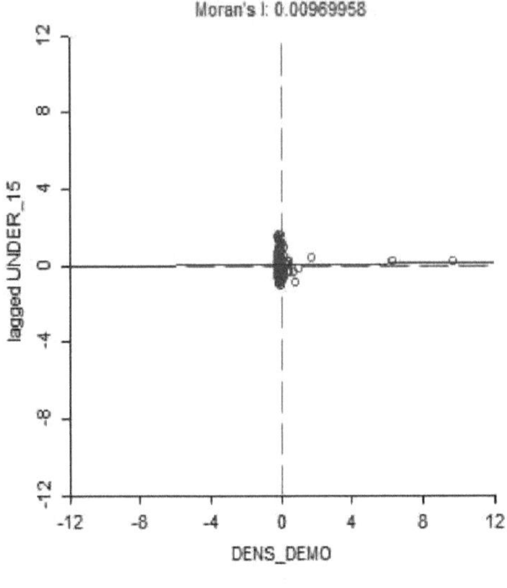

p = 0.365 (Not significant).

Figure 6. Moran's scatter diagram (bivariate analysis). Analysis of the socioeconomic and demographic variables of the patient's city of residence (X axis) and the weighted average morbidity rate of neighbouring cities (Y axis). A) Illiteracy rate. B) Gini Index. C) Illiteracy rate. D) Demographic density.

Moran's scatter diagrams of the socio-demographic variables income and population density showed spatial independence. These, at least at first glance, are not in line with the epidemiological outline that they can affect and/or predispose a given population to developing leprosy. These variables showed negative spatial auto-correlation, which further encourages discussions about the main factors that may be affecting the state of Mato Grosso in order to maximise the statistics.

However, the illiteracy rate and Gini Coefficient variables showed a positive spatial auto-correlation, indicating that these two factors influence the process of misinformation and social inequality, thus contributing to predisposing a certain population to the risk of falling ill. (SIMÕES; DELELLO, 2005) proved in their study that the socioeconomic profile of the sample studied was predominantly concentrated among the less privileged strata of society.

In a study of 61 people notified to the Leprosy Control Programme, 73.7% were male, which indicates a higher incidence among men, as has already been shown in other studies. This investigation found a high percentage of illiterate people, a situation that was more prevalent among women, which reinforces the idea that the disease affects people with a low level of education more, a fact that can reduce the opportunity to access information about health and illness (SOBRINHO; MATHIAS; LINCOLN, 2009).

Araújo (2003) encourages these discussions in his work, pointing out that although leprosy is still prevalent in the poorest countries and in the least favoured strata of the population, the weight of variables such as housing, nutritional status, concomitant infections (HIV and malaria) and previous infections with other mycobacteria is not known for sure. The role of genetic factors has long been evaluated, and the distribution of the disease in clusters, families or communities with a common genetic background suggests this possibility.

Why does leprosy become endemic in some areas, despite intense efforts to combat it? Are there geographic, socio-cultural or economic dynamics and flow and occupation factors influencing the permanent circulation of the bacillus in the population? Could the proximity of people living in areas of high population density be an aggravating factor? Subclinical infection could be a source of hidden transmission, acting as a perpetuator of the endemic (DUARTE-CUNHA, 2012).

It's interesting how these variables are found in the literature almost homogeneously as predisposing factors. Even though the preliminary information from the diagrams did not show a positive spatial autocorrelation, it would not be sensible to make assertions about this data. This position is in line with (AMARAL; LANA, 2008) who report that socio-economic and cultural conditions have a major influence on the distribution and spread of the leprosy endemic, with a close link to precarious housing conditions, low schooling and migratory movements that facilitate the spread of the disease. In endemic countries, there are differences in prevalence between regions, states, micro-regions, municipalities and, in the case of large cities, between inter-urban spaces, concentrating in places of great poverty.

On the other hand, the same authors emphasise that the relationship between leprosy and social conditions needs to be further explored in order to establish links between them.

Ribeiro (2009) reports that despite recent discoveries about the genetic component involved in the development of leprosy, socio-economic and environmental factors cannot be excluded in determining the disease, nor can the actions to combat and control it proposed by the World Health Organisation (WHO) and the Ministry of Health be relegated to the background, since these are issues of paramount importance in reversing the current epidemiological profile of leprosy in Brazil and important for achieving the goal of eliminating the disease proposed by the WHO, which is a prevalence of less than one case per 10,000 inhabitants.

However, Vieira et al (2008) insist that in most regions of the world the incidence of the disease is higher in men than in women. There are other factors that favour endemicity, such as unfavourable socio-economic conditions, precarious living and health conditions, and the large number of people living in the same environment, all of which influence the risk of falling ill.

In this context, it is pertinent to think about other possibilities of contamination and/or other predisposing factors that may be directly linked to the vulnerability of certain regions, providing daily contact with products that in the long term are tangible factors in the transmission of mycobacteria. (SOUZA, 2012) emphasises that the main source of infection and reservoir is man, but the disease is not exclusive to humans. The significance of other sources of infection and natural reservoirs has not been fully elucidated, although there is knowledge about some of their potential in the transmission of leprosy.

In addition to individual immunological conditions, (OPROMOLLA; DALBEN; CARDIM; 2006) other factors influence the risk of falling ill with leprosy. These include those related to endemic levels and unfavourable socio-economic conditions, such as poor living and health conditions and the large number of people living in the same environment. Knowing the living and health conditions of the various population groups is an indispensable stage in the process of planning the provision of services and evaluating the impact of health actions.

Alencar et al (2008) reveals that some studies carried out in the north-eastern region of Brazil, specifically in Ceará, have contributed to a greater understanding of this aspect of the epidemiology of the disease. Municipalities with greater social inequality had the highest leprosy detection and prevalence coefficients, reinforcing the fact that socioeconomic and environmental indicators are also important predictors of leprosy.

According to Souza (2012), the bacillus has been shown to be present in the water, food and milk of mothers with leprosy, but there is no direct evidence of transmission of the disease through ingestion.

Putting other possibilities on the table to justify the high prevalence rates of leprosy in the state of Mato Grosso is an appropriate approach to the statistics and behaviour of the disease at the federal unit level. Considering that the socio-demographic variables showed spatial independence in Moran's scatter diagram, what other factors could be directly involved in the process of these patients falling ill? And with regard to children under fifteen, considering the migration process and the long incubation period of the disease, what predisposing factors could be associated? Along these lines, (SOUZA, 2012) reports that some authors have mentioned that specific antigens of non-cultivable mycobacteria have been found in soil, vegetation and water samples, the inoculation of which in animals has reproduced a disease similar to leprosy in humans. In Indonesia, water contamination by M. Leprae and a higher prevalence of leprosy among individuals who used contaminated water for drinking has been demonstrated in endemic places.

Ferreira, Ignotti and Gamba (2011) maintain a cautious stance, arguing that the importance of the influence of unfavourable socioeconomic conditions related to a higher risk of falling ill on leprosy transmission has been discussed in other studies. Unfavourable socio-economic conditions combined with the precarious housing conditions to which these individuals are exposed and the immune response to Mycobacterium leprae could favour the recurrence of the disease.

CHAPTER 10

CONCLUSION

In this study on the behaviour of leprosy in the state of Mato Grosso, it was decided to take a spatial approach over a five-year time series in order to observe the past behaviour of this pathology in all of the state's municipalities. Leprosy is a disease without borders, which has historically spread across the globe through extrinsic factors such as wars, agglomerations, poverty and high migratory flows.

Mato Grosso is a state on the rise, both economically and politically. Its vast and eclectic demography allows it to expand its potential. Paradoxically, it borders states that are hyperendemic for leprosy, such as Tocantis, Pará and Amazonas. Despite the positive factors of its economy, it is imperative to emphasise that from a geographical point of view, the state of Mato Grosso is vulnerable to the continuous and persistent transmission of the etiological agent of Hansen's disease in its domains.

This introduction was corroborated by the geospatial analysis carried out in this research, which clearly showed that all 141 municipalities in the state have incidence and prevalence coefficients above national and international recommendations. Of course, the magnitude of the prevalence was greater in areas with an extensive territory. At this point, it should be realised that the current migratory flow acts in a synergistic and heterogeneous way within the vulnerability aspects of a given population and/or community.

Another crucial factor that should be mentioned is the current importance of health information systems. These, although they have their operational biases, have made a significant contribution to adequately measuring the entire flow of information from the network and programmes, such as SINAN and DATASUS. Through them, it is possible to know the real epidemiological situation.

The results of the study also showed that the rates of leprosy in children under fifteen in Mato Grosso were worrying, although in line with the literature and the organisations responsible. The univariate analysis for morbidity showed spatial significance, suggesting that municipalities with high rates of the disease are surrounded by areas that are also contaminated.
Based on this premise, it is likely that there are foci of transmission of the multibacillary forms circulating among them. Considering the incubation period and the close and prolonged inter-human contact, this gives rise to the idea that there are still a large number of undiagnosed and untreated cases.

With regard to socioeconomic and demographic variables, the results were not homogeneous. The income factor and demographic density resulted in spatial independence, not demonstrating in this study that these two factors are relevant in terms of predisposition to the future development of leprosy.

A positive spatial association was observed for the illiteracy rate and the gini coefficient as predictors of situations of vulnerability. People with low access to information are considered a risk group by the Ministry. In leprosy, the information factor is crucial. Even though leprosy is not a lethal disease, patients who receive early diagnosis and subsequent treatment with MDT have a lower chance of neuritis, reactions and sequelae. Unfortunately, Mato Grosso has a large number of municipalities that are geographically distant from reference centres, another complicating factor.

Regardless, information is vital for patients to understand that their signs and symptoms may be related to leprosy, leading them to quickly seek out a health centre. It should be added here that there are still people who don't seek care even though they have the information, but for reasons of stigma, prejudice and fear.

Social inequalities are a reality in Brazil, an underdeveloped country with different geographical, political and economic characteristics. This problem leads a portion of society to live on an income that is not appropriate, allowing families and/or communities to live in areas without the minimum health conditions, such as basic sanitation, leisure, school, work and housing.

This research was satisfactory, but even given the results, other questions arise. What are the factors that lead to these high rates of leprosy in Mato Grosso? Are there other factors that are contributing to the high rates of leprosy in children under fifteen? If so, which ones? Is the Hansen's bacillus present in the soil, water and breast milk to the extent that it maximises the development of the disease in the long term? To what extent can the state's border regions be held responsible? What other factors intrinsic to the geographical limits of the state of Mato Grosso may be contributing to this epidemiology.

It is also important to note that the various studies carried out in this area in recent years have helped to better characterise the behaviour of this disease in the federal units, breaking down previous paradigms and bringing up current and relevant issues that deserve to be discussed and taken forward by professionals, managers, technical teams and the bodies responsible.

REFERENCES

ALENCAR CHM et al. Leprosy in the municipality of Fortaleza, CE, Brazil: epidemiological and operational aspects in children under 15 (1995-2006). **Rev Bras Enferm**, Brasília 2008; 61(esp): 694-700.

ALVES CJM et al. **Evaluation of the degree of disability of patients diagnosed with leprosy in a Dermatology Service in the State of São Paulo**. Bauru: [s.n], 2010.

AMARAL EP, LANA FCF. Spatial analysis of leprosy in the micro-region of Almenara, MG. **Rev Bras Enferm.** Brasília, 2008; 61(esp): 701-7.

AMARAL RCO. **Sensory and motor evaluation of leprosy neuritis patients submitted to neurolysis in the state of Rondônia** between 2000 and 2003. Brasília: University of Brasília, 2006. Dissertation, 128 p.

AMARAL EFL. **Building and understanding tables**. Available at: < http://www.ernestoamaral.com/docs/dcp033-101/Aulas27-28.pdf> Accessed on 17 December 2013.

ANDRADE L. **Analysis of the spatial distribution of juvenile homicides in a Brazilian triple border municipality between 2000 and 2007**. Dissertation. State University of Maringá. Postgraduate Programme in Nursing. Master's Degree in Nursing. Maringá, 2009.

ARAÚJO MG. **Leprosy in Brazil.** Belo Horizonte: [s.n], 2003.

BARBIERI CLA, MARQUES HHS. **Leprosy in children and adolescents: literature review and current situation in Brazil**. Pediatrics (São Paulo) 2009; 31(4):281-90.

BOTI NCL, AQUINO KAA. Veganin's Way of the Cross of Leprosy. **Rev Bras Enferm**, 61 (esp): 676 - 81, 2008.

BRAZIL. Ministry of Health. Health Policy Secretariat. Department of Primary Care. **Guide to leprosy control**. 3 ed. Brasília: [s.n], 2002.

BRAZIL. Ministry of Health. Health Policy Secretariat. Department of Primary Care. **Dermatology in Primary Care**. 1 ed. Brasília: [s.n], 2002.

BRAZIL. Ministry of Health. Health Surveillance Secretariat. Department of Epidemiological Surveillance. **Corticosteroids in leprosy**. Brasília: [s.n], 2010.

BRAZIL. Ministry of Health. Health Surveillance Secretariat. Department of Epidemiological Surveillance. **Leprosy and Human Rights: rights and duties of SUS users**. Brasília: [s.n], 2008.

BRAZIL. Ministry of Health. Health Surveillance Secretariat. General Coordination of the National Leprosy Control Programme. **Epidemiological Situation in Brazil and the World**. Brasília, 2010.

BRAZIL. Ministry of Health. Health Surveillance Secretariat. Department of Epidemiological Surveillance. **Guide to Technical Procedures: bacilloscopy in leprosy**. Brasília: [s.n], 2010.

BRAZIL. Ministry of Health. Health Surveillance Secretariat. Department of Epidemiological Surveillance. **Leprosy Epidemiological Situation**. Brasília: [s.n], 2011.

BRAZIL. Ministry of Health. Health Surveillance Secretariat. **Department of Communicable Disease Surveillance.** Integrated Strategic Action Plan. Brasília, 2012.

BRAZIL. PortalBrasil . Disponívelem :< http://www.brasil.gov.br/saude/2012/10/casos-de-hanseniase-diminuiram-26-nos- ultimos-10-anos> Accessed 09 December 2013.

BRAZIL SCHOOL. **Aspects of the population of Mato Grosso**. Available at: <http://www.brasilescola.com/brasil/aspectos-populacao-mato-grosso.htm> Accessed on 17December2013 .

BRAZIL. Leprosy Control Programme. Leprosy Epidemiological Surveillance Division. State Department of Health. **Leprosy Epidemiological Situation**. Brasília, 2011.

BRAZIL. Ministry of Health. Health Surveillance. Surveillance Department Available at :< http://portalsaude.saude.gov.br/portalsaude/noticia/4085/162/novos-casos-de- hanseniase-caem-15-em-um-ano.html>. Accessed on 10/04/2012.

BRAZIL. Health Surveillance Secretariat. Department of Epidemiological Surveillance. **Epidemiological situation of leprosy in Brazil - analysis of selected indicators in the last decade and challenges for elimination.** Vol 44, n° 11. Brasília, 2013.

DESSUNTI EM et al. Leprosy: the control of contacts in the municipality of Londrina- PR in a period of ten years. **Rev Bras Enferm**, 61(esp): 689 - 93. Brasília, 2008.

CUIABÁ DAILY. **Inequality and poverty in Mato Grosso**. Available at:< http://www.diariodecuiaba.com.br/detalhe.php?cod=341469> Accessed 17 December 2013.

DUARTE-CUNHA M et al. Epidemiological aspects of leprosy: a spatial approach. **Cad. Saúde Pública**. 28(6):1143-1155. Rio de Janeiro, 2012.

EIDT LM. A brief history of leprosy: its expansion from the world to the Americas, Brazil and Rio Grande do Sul and its trajectory in Brazilian public health. **Saúde e Sociedade** v.13, n.2, p.76-88, May/Aug, 2004.

FERREIRA SMB, IGNOTTI E, GAMBA MA. Factors associated with leprosy relapse in Mato Grosso. **Rev Saúde Pública,** 2011. 45(4):756-64.

FERREIRA IN, ALVAREZ RRA. Leprosy in children under fifteen in the municipality of Paracatu-MG. **Rev Bras Epidemiol.** 8(1): 41-9, 2005.

FERREIRA MAA, ANTUNES CMF. Factors associated with ML Flow seropositivity in patients and contacts of leprosy patients under 18 years of age. **Journal of the Brazilian Society of Tropical Medicine,** 2008. 41(Supplement II): 60-66.

FOSS NT. Immunological aspects of leprosy. **Medicina, Ribeirão Preto, 30:** 335-339, Jul/Sep 1997.

GARCIA DR et al. Spatial analysis of leprosy cases, focusing on the risk area, in a basic health unit in the municipality of Cáceres (MT). **Cad. Saúde Colet**. Rio de Janeiro, 2013. 21 (2): 168-72

GOVERNMENT OF THE STATE OF MATO GROSSO. **Information about Mato Grosso**. Available at: <www.cidades.com.br/estado/mato grosso/mt.html> Accessed on 05 May 2013.

GOULART IMB, PENNA GO, CUNHA G. Immunopathology of leprosy: the complexity of the mechanisms of the host immune response to Mycobacterium Leprae. **Revista da Sociedade Brasileira de Medicina Tropical** 35(4): 365-375, Jul/Aug, 2002.

IMBIRIBA EB et al. Epidemiological profile of leprosy in children under fifteen years of age, Manaus (AM), 1998-2005. **Rev Saúde Pública**, 2008. 42(6):1021-6.

LANNA FCF et al. Leprosy in children under 15 in the Jequitinhonha Valley, Minas Gerais. **Rev. bras. enferm.** Brasília, 2007. 60(6): 696-700.

LEITE VMC, LIMA JWO, GONÇALVES HS. Silent neuropathy in leprosy patients in the city of Fortaleza, Ceará, Brazil. **Cad. Saúde Pública**: Rio de Janeiro, 2011. 27(4):659-665.

LIMA LS et al. Clinical-epidemiological characterisation of patients diagnosed with leprosy in the municipality of Caxias, MA. **Rev Bras Clin Med**, 2009;7:74-83.

MAINENTI DAM. **Implementation of Process Management in a National Reference Centre in Brazil: impact on disability prevention.** Master's dissertation. University of Uberlândia, Minas Gerais, Brazil, 2010.

MAGALHÃES MCC et al. Migration and Leprosy in Mato Grosso. Executive Secretariat of the Ministry of Health - Brasília (DF), Brazil Department of Geography of the University of São Paulo - São Paulo (SP), State Secretariat of Health of Mato Grosso - Cuiabá (MS), Department of Community Health of the Faculty of Medicine of the Federal University of Ceará - Fortaleza (CE). **Rev Bras Epidemiol**, 2011. 14(3): 386-97.

MBI. Geographical coordinates of the state of Mato Grosso. Available at: <www.mbi.com.br/mbi/biblioteca/utilidades/dddcepmt/> Accessed on 04 May 2013.

MELÃO S et al. Epidemiological profile of leprosy patients in the extreme south of Santa Catarina, from 2001 to 2007. **Journal of the Brazilian Society of**

Tropical Medicine . 44(1):79-84, jan/fev, 2011.

MENDONÇA VA et al. Immunology of Leprosy. Belo Horizonte: Federal University of Minas Gerais. **An Bras Dermatol.** 2008;83(4):343-50.

MOSCHIONI C. **Risk factors for physical disability recorded at the time of diagnosis of 19,283 new cases of leprosy between 2000 and 2005 in Minas Gerais.** Dissertation (Master's Degree in Health Sciences: Infectious Diseases and Tropical Medicine). UFMG School of Medicine. Belo Horizonte, 2007.

Monot M et al. On the Origin of Leprosy. **Science** 308: 1040-1042 (2005)

NOGUEIRA W et al. **Perspectivas de Eliminação da Hanseníase**. São Paulo. **Hansen. Int.**, 210(1):19-28. 1995.

OLIVEIRA CAR. de. **Epidemiological profile of leprosy in children under fifteen in the municipality of Teresina**. Master's thesis. Fiocruz. Oswaldo Cruz Foundation. National School of Public Health. Teresina, 2008.

WHO. World Health Organisation. **Global Strategy to Alleviate the Burden of Leprosy and Sustain Leprosy Control Activities**, Plan:2006-2010, Geneva, 2005.

PAHO. World Health Organisation. **Elimination of Leprosy in the Americas**. Brasilia, 2002.

OPROMOLLA DVA, BACCARELLI R. **Prevention of Disabilities and Rehabilitation in Leprosy.** Lauro de Souza Lima Institute: Bauru, 2003.

OPROMOLLA PA, DALBEN I, CARDIM M. Geostatistical analysis of leprosy cases in the State of São Paulo, 1991-2002. **Rev Saúde Pública**, 2006. 40(5):907-13.

OPROMOLLA DVA. **Notions of Hansenology**. Bauru, 2000.

PAES ALV et al. Clinical and epidemiological profile of leprosy patients. Belém- PA, 2011. **Rev. para. Med** 24(3/4), Jul/Dec. 2010.

PEDRO HSP et al. Leprosy: Comparison between the operational classification in the Notifiable Diseases Information System and the result of bacilloscopy.
Hansen Int 2009; 34(2): 13-19.

PEROBELLI FS, HADDAD EA. Patterns of interstate trade in Brazil, 1985 and 1997. **Rev. econ. contemp**. Rio de Janeiro, v.10, n.1, p. 61-88, apr. 2006.

PIMENTEL MIF et al. Silent neuritis in multibacillary leprosy assessed through the evolution of disabilities before, during or after multidrug therapy. **An bras Dermatol**, Rio de Janeiro, 79(2):169-179, Mar/Apr 2004.

PINTO RA. Clinical and epidemiological profile of patients reported with leprosy in a specialised hospital in Salvador, Bahia. **Rev B.S.Publica Miolo**. V 34, n° 4.

PIRES CAA et al. Leprosy in children under fifteen: the importance of contact examination. **Rev Paul Pediatr** 2012. 30(2):292-5.

Ponte KMA, Ximenes Neto FRG. Leprosy: the reality for adolescents. **Rev Bras Enferm** 2005 May/Jun; 58(3):296-301.

PORTALMATOGROSSO . Available at : <http://mteseusmunicipios.com.br/NG/conteudo.php?cid= 13557&sid=44> *Accessed 17 December 2013.*

QUEIROZ ML. **Leprosy in the state of Mato Grosso**. Master's thesis. Federal University of Mato Grosso. Institute of Collective Health. Cuiabá, 2009.

QUEIROZ MS, PUNTEL MA. ***The leprosy epidemic:*** **an ultidiscillinary perspective** [online]. Rio de Janeiro: FIOCRUZ, 1997. 120 p

RIBEIRO IT. **LEPROSY IN THE CURRENT EPIDEMIOLOGICAL CONTEXT: BASES FOR CONTROLLING THE ENDEMIC**. Final Coursework (Postgraduate). Castelo Branco University. Campinas, 2009.

RIDLEY DS, JOPLING WH. **Classification of leprosy according to immunity**. A five-group system. Int. J. Lepr. Other Mycobact. Dis. 34(3), 255-273.

ROMÃO ER, MAZZONI AM. Epidemiological profile of leprosy in the municipality of Guarulhos, SP. **Rev Eidemiol Control Infect**.;3(1):22-27, 2013.

RIVITTI S, SAMPAIO SAP. **Dermatology**. 3 ed. São Paulo: Artes Médicas, 2007.

SANTOS AS, CASTRO DS, FALQUETO, A. Risk factors for leprosy transmission. **Rev Bras Enferm**: Brasília, 2008. 61(esp): 738-43.

SANTOS AE, RODRIGUES AL, LOPES DL. **Applications of Empirical Bayesian Estimators for Spatial Analysis of Mortality Rates**. Department of Statistics - Federal University of Minas Gerais. Belo Horizonte, 2005.

SIMÕES MJS, DELELLO D. Estudo do comportamento social dos pacientes de hanseníase do município de São Carlos-SP. **Revista Espaço para a Saúde, Londrina,** v.7 ,n.1, p.10-15 , dez.2005.

SOBRINHO RSS. **Epidemiological profile of leprosy in the state of Paraná during the elimination period**. Master's dissertation. University of Maringá. Paraná. Brazil, 2007.

SOBRINHO RAS, MATHIAS, TAF, LINCOLN PB. Profile of leprosy cases notified in the 14ª Regional Health Department of Paraná after decentralisation of the programme to the municipal level. **Cienc Cuid Saude** 2009 Jan/Mar; 8(1):19-26.

BRAZILIAN SOCIETY OF HANSENOLOGY and BRAZILIAN SOCIETY OF DERMATOLOGY. Guidelines Project. **Leprosy: Reactive Episodes**, 2003

BRAZILIAN SOCIETY OF DERMATOLOGY. Portal of the Brazilian Society of Dermatology. **Against Leprosy**. Available at :< http://www.sbd.org.br/campanha/hanseniase/MSaude.aspx> Accessed 09 December 2013.

BRAZILIAN SOCIETY OF LEPROSY. BRAZILIAN ACADEMY OF NEUROLOGY. BRAZILIAN SOCIETY OF CLINICAL NEUROPHYSIOLOGY. Guidelines Project. Leprosy: **Diagnosis and Treatment of Neuropathy**, 2003.

SOUZA CS. **Leprosy: Clinical forms and differential diagnosis.** Ribeirão Preto, 30: 325-334, jul/set. 1997

SOUZA LR. **Social conditioning factors in the delimitation of leprosy endemic areas.** Thesis (Doctorate) Faculty of Medicine, University of São Paulo. Preventive Medicine Programme.

SOUZA LWF. Leprosy reactions in patients discharged from hospital after cure by multidrug therapy. **Revista da Sociedade Brasileira de Medicina Tropical.** 43(6):737-739,nov/dez,2010.

GEOGRAPHY ONLY. Map of the State of Mato Grosso. Available at: <www.sogeografia.com.br/Conteudos/GeografiaFisica/Cartografia> Accessed on 03 May 2013.

TEIXEIRA MAG. SILVEIRA VM. FRANÇA ER. Epidemiological and clinical characteristics of leprosy reactions in paucibacillary and multibacillary individuals treated at two reference centres for leprosy in the city of Recife, state of Pernambuco. **Revista da Sociedade Brasileira de Medicina Tropical** 43(3):287-292, mai/jun, 2010.

VERONESI R, FOCACCIA R. **Tratado de Infectologia**. 4 ed. São Paulo: Atheneu, 2009.

VIEIRA CS et al. Evaluation and Control of Missing Contacts of Leprosy Patients. **Rev Bras Enferm**, 61(esp): 682 - 8. Brasília, 2008.

VIEIRA CK, REMACRE AZ. **BIVARIATE ANALYSIS: AN EXPERIMENTAL CONDITIONAL HOPE APPROACH.** Available at: < **http://www.prp.rei.unicamp.br/pibic/congressos/ixcongresso/cdrom/pdfN/486.p df**> Accessed 17 December 2013.

Yawalker SJ. **Leprosy.** 2 ed. Novartis, 2002.

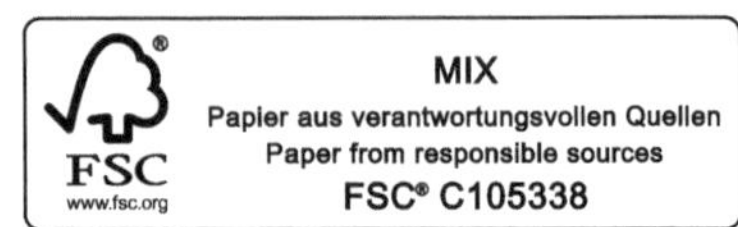

Printed by Books on Demand GmbH, Norderstedt / Germany